The South African women's guide to
SELF-DEFENCE

Sanette Smit

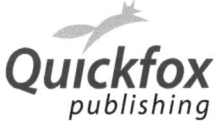

Published by Quickfox Publishing
PO Box 50660 West Beach 7449
Cape Town, South Africa
www.quickfox.co.za | info@quickfox.co.za

THE SOUTH AFRICAN WOMEN'S GUIDE TO SELF-DEFENCE

Third edition 2021
ISBN: 978-1-920-70070-6

Copyright © 2021 Sanette Smit

All rights reserved. No part of this publication may be reproduced, stored in a retrieval system, or transmitted, in any form or by any means, without the prior written permission of the publisher.

Editor – Joy Clack
Photographer – Pieter Smit
Proofreader – Proofread cc and Quickfox Publishing
Typesetting and production – Quickfox Publishing
Printing – Print-on-Demand, Cape Town

CONTENTS

Preface 11
Introduction 15

1 BACKGROUND ON RAPE 19

2 PATTERNS OF RAPE 30
    Confidence rape 31
    Blitz rape 34
    Anger rape 36
    Power rape 37
    Fantasy rape 39
    Date rape 41
    Gang rape 42
    Convenience rape 44
    Sadistic rape (organized and disorganized) 45
    Styles of attack 46

3 DYNAMICS OF SELF-DEFENCE 47
    Your attitude 52
    Physical considerations 57

4 BODY TARGET AREAS 68
    Body from the back 69
    Body from the front 70

5 BASIC SELF-DEFENCE TECHNIQUES 71

Introduction 71
Hand and arm techniques to the face and neck........................... 80
Hand and arm techniques to the front of the body..................... 87
Hand and arm techniques to the back of the body 90
Wrist and special hand techniques... 91
Kicking and leg techniques... 92

6 SELF-DEFENCE SCENARIOS 96

Attacks from the front.. 97
   Attack to the throat with both hands (1)............................... 97
   Attack to the throat with both hands (2)............................. 100
   Attack to the throat with one hand (1)................................ 103
   Attack to the throat with one hand (2)................................ 105
   Attack to the throat with one hand (3)................................ 107
   Wrist-grab with one hand (1).. 110
   Wrist-grab with one hand (2).. 113
General attacks to the face... 115
General attack from the front.. 117
Attacks from behind... 120
   Attack from behind with one arm around the throat 120
   Bear-hug (1)... 122
   Bear-hug (2)... 125
   Mouth and waist grip... 128
   Armlock attack with both hands 132
   Hair grab from behind 134
   Single-arm grip around the throat...................................... 135

- Attacks from the side 138
  - *Stranglehold with one arm around the neck (1)* 138
  - *Stranglehold with one arm around the neck (2)* 140
  - *Stranglehold with one arm around the neck (3)* 142
  - *Attack to the throat with both hands* 144
- Attack while sitting down 146
- Attacks on the ground and lying down 147
  - *Attack to the body with both hands* 147
  - *Attack to the throat with both hands (1)* 150
  - *Attack to the throat with both hands (2)* 152
  - *Attack to the throat with both hands (3)* 155
  - *General ground technique (1)* 159
  - *General ground technique (2)* 162
  - *General ground technique (3)* 163
  - *Getting up off the ground* 164

7 OBJECTS AS WEAPONS **168**

Acknowledgments 170
Resources 172

From the desk of Rape Crisis

The South African Police Service reported that 55 114 women reported rape between April 2004 and March 2005 in South Africa. This report is confined to the narrow definition of rape and does not include other forms of rape such as anal rape, oral rape, rape with an object and male rape. Rape Crisis and other organisations who deal with sexual violence believe that only one in nine rape survivors report rape in South Africa on an annual basis and no-one really knows what the real situation is.

We live in a country that is guided by a progressive Constitution and a Bill of Rights, but this protection is hampered by the fact that we continue to live in a patriarchal society that reinforces accepted gender stereotypes and the myths and perceptions around rape. The reality of this is that these myths and perceptions undermine the credibility of survivors; society places the responsibility for the rape onto a survivor. It is unacceptable that our country has some of the highest levels of rape and gender-based violence in the world, and the time has come for women and men to take collective responsibility to end the scourge of violence against women and ensure that women are free. To achieve significant change, there needs to be a fundamental shift in attitudes and behavior, which will take time.

While we work towards this change, women are encouraged to empower themselves. The one thing we *can* do is to become aware of how to prevent rape and assault happening to us as individuals. Sanette Smit has a passion for empowering women to take control, make informed choices and become aware of how to defend themselves in various situations. This valuable book is not about stopping rape and it does not guarantee anything, but it will help you become more aware and provide you with the knowledge and the ability to reduce your risks of being raped.

We encourage all South Africans to empower themselves and join the movement to end rape and violence against women.

Chantel Cooper
Past director, Rape Crisis Cape Town
From the diary of a rape survivor...

I watched Smitti and her trainees re-enact my rape scene – small girls fighting off the huge colonel that volunteered to play the role of the attacker.

If only.

If only I had known these few basic self-defence techniques, I would not have had to face the pain, the emotions, the nausea, the rage, the fear, the sadness, and the repugnance.

Although I fought my rapist (and I fought him hard), he got the better of me. He raped me, he cut me, he tied me up and left me for dead.

If only.

To feel a strange man insert his penis into me against my will is probably one of the worst moments of my life. He hurt me physically, he broke my teeth, and he stabbed me in the face, neck, ears and arms. But worse, he raped me.

I stopped fighting at the point when he held a broken glass to my stomach. Rather than let him cut and kill me, I gave in to him.

If only.

If only I had known one or two easy manoeuvres to use at this point when he was at his most vulnerable. If only I had known a movement to stop this madman when he silently came up behind me, holding a screwdriver to my neck.

If only I had met Smitti before I had to face this nightmare.

Smitti never once said – if you had studied karate or self-defence you would have been okay. She said that it was great that I had the courage to fight and that she admired me for my strength.

I survived the trauma of rape. I survived due to the support of family and friends and strangers who became friends. People, amongst many, many others, people like Smitti.

But none of us will ever be quite the same again.

Lois Wagner
Survived rape of 30 December 1995
From the heart of a rape survivor…

One glorious afternoon in October 1994 on an idyllic beach in the Seychelles, a stranger raped me. He violently attacked me, threatened to kill me, tried to strangle me with my T-shirt and shoved handfuls of sand into my mouth to prevent me from making a noise. Shock numbed me to my bones yet my mind remained alert. Having no knowledge of self-defence, I knew that if I wanted to survive the attack, I would have to remain calm and obey his orders. I chose to react in this way and to pray while he raped me. Within seconds he stopped, withdrew and retreated, still threatening to kill me as he left the scene.

I did what I thought was best in the situation in which I found myself. For other women faced with the same situation, knowledge of self-defence would be a life saver. However, women should not set themselves up to think that they are invincible. Self-defence training should not create a false sense of security, but rather a heightened sense of awareness.

After attending one of Smitti's brilliant self-defence workshops in 2002, I felt empowered as a woman, more aware and more confident in averting certain dangerous situations. I felt better able to defend myself should another attack arise. While teaching self-defence, Smitti reminds women of their inner strength and beauty, and urges them to realize their powers and identify those important intuitive feelings that they so often ignore.

I have always known that the rape is not my fault, that I am stronger and more powerful than a rapist, that I have nothing to be ashamed of, that I am well and he is ill. Very few rape survivors feel this way and over the years I have come to realize that my purpose is to speak out against rape, and to support and empower other rape survivors.

Those who know me love me unconditionally, respect me, and accept and believe my story. Their love and amazing support, coupled with my ongoing involvement with other rape survivors and rape-related work, has been invaluable in my recovery.

Kathy Rath
Rape survivor, Port Elizabeth
From Smitti's right hand...

When Smitti (Sanette) invited me to help make her dream of writing a self-defence book a reality, I was both excited and nervous. Excited, because I totally believe in her work and what she is trying to achieve in terms of empowering and encouraging women to acknowledge their own capabilities, beauty and strength. Nervous, because I hoped that I would be able to do her the justice she deserves in accurately capturing, in words, the essence, dynamism, energy and passion for her work that she expresses in a very physical and demonstrative manner, every day.

This book has been based on Smitti's more than forty years of experience in the art of defence and, more specifically, self-defence. It is the result of her extensive studies on rape, interviews with countless rape survivors, research on rapists, and hands-on experience teaching karate and then self-defence to a few hundred thousand women and girls.

I feel honoured to be a part of this book and have no doubt that you will benefit, as I have, from the valuable information contained within its pages and from the inspiration and motivation of one of the most dynamic women I know.

Vanessa Wilson

PREFACE

While I have always been concerned about the dangers facing women regarding physical violence and rape, it was only when I was researching the subject of rape for my 3rd Dan Black Belt study piece that I became truly aware of, and utterly horrified by, the alarming statistics of rape and severe brutality of some of these cases. What horrified me more was the fact that very few people seemed concerned about it and that most were victims of the myths and misconceptions about rape that have continually served to disempower and harm women.

One of the great myths of rape – that women have 'asked for it' by way of dress and behavior – has placed the shame and responsibility of rape squarely on the victims' shoulders, so much so that many rape survivors choose not to disclose details of their rape to either the authorities or those closest to them for fear of rejection and contempt. This myth has also resulted in complacency on the part of the authorities and courts when it comes to prosecuting rape. In other words, rape has never been taken seriously enough and, in many instances, is still 'conveniently' swept under the carpet.

Sadly, women have also unwittingly contributed to the myths of rape by failing to use the opportunities presented to them to put right some of these misconceptions. An ignorant comment such as 'she was a fool to walk around so late at night – she asked for it!', is a perfect opportunity for us to educate those who clearly do not know better. The reality is that a high proportion of rape actually occurs in a woman's home where she thinks she's safe! Yet, how many of us actually have the courage to rise to this challenge?

While attitudes to rape have changed dramatically over the past few years and more and more women are coming forward and reporting incidences of rape to the police – thanks in part to uprisings of women in the fight against Gender Based Violence (GBV) and the global #MeToo movement – we find that we are still fighting a tremendously inefficient legal system and, of course, centuries of sexist attitudes towards women.

It is only more recently that we have seen certain structures being formed to give rape more attention. Police are receiving special training in how to work with women who have been raped, and an increasing number of centres are being established for post-rape counselling. This is a start, but not nearly good enough to deal with a crisis that has grown out-of-hand. It has become clear to many that the only protection we really have against rape is to be found in rape prevention education and effective self-defence training. To keep women as safe as possible, we must strive to empower women as individuals – mentally and physically. Since 90% of women are attacked when they are alone, it is important that they adopt a proactive attitude and learn to rely on themselves for their protection. It is not enough to wait for society or culture to change to get the help they need.

I believe that rape prevention education and training should be implemented at school level. In fact, we should seriously consider making it part of the school curriculum so that we can create a sustainable level of awareness and enable children to develop appropriate self-defence skills and an attitude that supports applying those skills when needed.

Yes, there is something women can do to drastically increase their chances of preventing a rape attack; and, no, women are not as weak and helpless as they think they are – they simply need to be taught *how* to defend themselves. This includes adopting the respective mind shift necessary for effective self-defence.

Strength does not necessarily win the battle. I have found this to be very true in more than 40 years of martial arts and self-defence training where I have witnessed women of differing physical capabilities successfully implement the self-defence techniques taught to them, against fellow male students.

It is important to understand, however, that there are situations in which self-defence would not be applicable, for various reasons. A woman's primary objective should be to get out of her particular situation alive, and she needs to make a judgement call based on her situation, mindset and skillset.

I believe that women who have had self-defence training have a very important and often underestimated weapon in an attack situation – the element of surprise. A would-be rapist rarely expects his victim to be armed with this kind of knowledge. Furthermore, self-defence training offers a woman many more options when dealing with an attack, and her chances of taking the right course of action in her attack situation are far greater. It's a pity that we do not hear enough about the successful cases where women have warded off a rape attack or life-threatening situation.

After carefully studying the rape statistics and increase in the crime rate in general in South Africa over the past 40 years, it is my opinion that we are fast approaching an era in which, by the time a woman has reached the age of 85, she will have been raped at least once. If she has not been raped, it will more than likely be due to one of the following two factors: either she was able to defend herself adequately, or she was fortunate enough to have had someone come to her assistance. Her escape from rape, however, will mean that another woman is raped twice!

One of the best self-defence tools a woman can use is the **power of intuition**. She has ready access to this wonderful gift – most men do not. Women should exercise, train and empower this ability. They should not ignore or doubt it, but should constantly seek to enhance and develop it. For example, how many women haven't experienced the feeling that their partners were having an affair? First, to have it denied, only to find out later that they were absolutely correct. Women are inclined to downplay that special sense of feeling because if they acknowledge what their intuition is telling them, they will have to do something about it, take responsibility, and this can be a scary thing for many of them.

Unfortunately, an attack situation forces women to face up to the responsibility, whether they like it or not, as ignoring it could mean the difference between life and death. By exercising intuition as a technique every day, a woman's awareness will be enhanced automatically in a natural way, making her much more likely to identify and avoid a potential threat before it's too late.

Although many of the principles and techniques shown in this book can be applied to a wide variety of attack scenarios, it is the one-on-one scenario with which we will concern ourselves. Situations involving more than one attacker or a weapon such as a gun are a lot more complex and require a greater degree of proficiency in the art of self-defence, both psychologically and physically.

I sincerely hope that this book benefits each and every person who reads it. It is more than just a practical book illustrating self-defence techniques – its purpose is to inspire, motivate and empower all women.

You are strong, you are wonderful, you deserve respect and love, and no one has the right to abuse you or rape you.

Believe and trust in yourself!

Sanette Smit

INTRODUCTION

Rape can happen to any woman, anywhere, and at any time – on her way home from work, at a night-club, while she is out jogging, at her office, even in her own home. Rape happens in all countries all over the world, within all races and at all levels of society. The violent act of rape knows no boundaries. Girls as young as 18 months and a woman as old as 114 years have been raped! No woman is safe from rape – all women are potential targets.

Rape is the single greatest threat to a woman and the effects of rape, especially brutal rape, can remain with a woman for life. Most women, either consciously or unconsciously, worry about being raped. While the long-term effects of rape are often difficult to measure, the immediate effects are a lot more obvious: many women experience withdrawal, lowered self-esteem, a decrease in self-confidence and morale, general mistrust, a deterioration in interpersonal relationships, even fear and guilt. Rape often affects not only the rape survivor/rape victim, but also family members, partners, friends and colleagues.

Rape statistics in South Africa

South Africa is reported as the country with the highest rape statistics in the world according to World Population Review 2020. A survey conducted by the SA Medical Research Council reveals that one in four South African men have admitted to committing rape.

In 2018/2019, the SAPS reported 52 420 cases of sexual offences, which equates to roughly 144 sexual offences daily. This is a gross misrepresentation as it is estimated that only one out of every nine offences in South Africa is reported. It is hard to know how many of these sexual offences refer specifically to rape, but according to the Institute for Security Studies, 56 272 rapes had been reported between the late 1990s and early 2000s. It is unlikely that the incidence of rape decreased from the early to late 2000s. It is more likely that fewer rapes were reported due to various factors, not least of which include a growing lack of trust in the police service and a poor conviction rate of only 7%, making women fearful for their future safety and unwilling to put themselves through the secondary trauma involved in seeing the process through to a less-than-desirable outcome. Other factors include current systems and attitudes, fear, humiliation, fear of loss of economic support by the abuser, intimidation by other family members, or because they know the rapist and fear being intimidated or further hurt by them. Unfortunatley, the systems required for collating data pertaining to rape and sexual abuse, the rapist, and the rape survivor, are still highly inadequate.

COMMON MISCONCEPTIONS ABOUT RAPE

- » Rape victims are sexy young women.
- » Nice women don't get raped.
- » Many rapes are instances in which a flirtatious woman changed her mind.
- » Jilted women make false accusations of rape.
- » Rape is primarily a sexual crime.
- » Women are 'asking for it' by their dress or actions.
- » It could never happen to me.
- » The rapist is a sex-starved deviant.
- » Women only get raped at night clubs and in dark alleys.
- » Women provoke men to rape them.
- » Only black men rape white women.

Rape – a woman's problem?

Society has made rape a woman's problem. Firstly, by blaming her for having been raped: 'What was she doing out at that time of night?', 'Her dress was too short', 'She accepted a date with him … what can she expect?' Secondly, by restricting her: 'Don't go out late at night', 'Don't drive alone', 'Lock your door and don't let anyone in.'

INTRODUCTION

It is rather ironic that women are stripped of their freedoms and privileges by the restrictions imposed on them, when men usually commit the crime of rape and for whom these restrictions would be most appropriate. It is also ironic that women are the ones taking responsibility for dealing with the rape issue when, again, it is men who are raping. Men should be sharing the responsibility for making our towns, cities and countries a safer place for all women. After all, these same women are their wives, girlfriends, sisters, mothers and daughters. Rape is very much a man's issue.

Because most men have chosen not to take responsibility for rape, women have had to become responsible for themselves. The legal system has never been of much assistance and, until fairly recently, neither have the police. Rapists have been caught, sometimes convicted, and then released on parole after having served minimum sentences. In most cases, these men have raped again.

Taking control

It is essential that we start taking control of our lives and safety. The threat of rape is all too real – more so now than ever before – and many women have come to realise the benefits of rape prevention awareness and self-defence as an aid to preventing rape. We should also be focusing on educating boys not to rape.

While nothing can guarantee your safety, awareness of rape prevention and a knowledge of effective self-defence techniques can drastically increase your chances of surviving and even preventing a rape attack. Through this education we can learn to fine-tune our skills, trust our intuition, increase our sense of awareness and project an aura of strength, confidence and positive attitude.

From a physical, self-defence point of view we can learn how to implement practical and effective self-defence techniques. This book will take you through the necessary steps for acquiring these skills. It will also provide valuable information about rape, the rapist, why rape happens, and the roles social upbringing, self-esteem and self-confidence have to play.

To achieve the full benefits of this book, it is suggested that all exercises be followed as directed. It is also beneficial to work with a partner wherever possible to enable you to physically 'try out' your techniques. In this way you will be able to gauge distance, proportion and power. It is also recommended that you attend a practical self-defence workshop at some point. More information on workshops is listed on page 172.

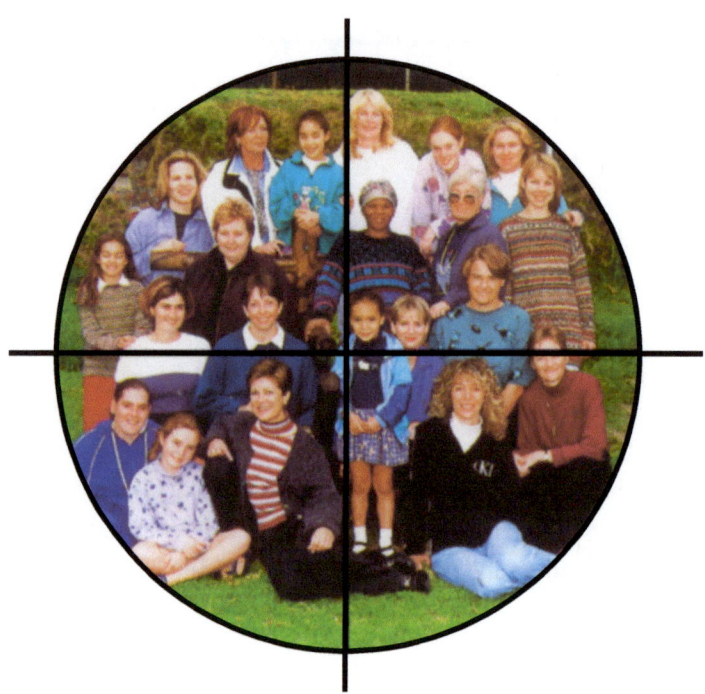

Every woman is a target!

1
BACKGROUND ON RAPE

What is rape?

The word 'rape' comes from the Latin *rapere*, which means 'to steal, seize or carry away'.

Although the statutes in different countries differ with regard to its legal definition, the definition of 'rape' in South Africa was amended in 2007 to include sexual penetration of any kind (not just with a penis) against the will or consent of the victim, even if the victim does not physically resist. Many women are afraid of resisting because they feel intimidated and fear being physically injured.

Rape Crisis, however, has a broader definition of rape. They think of rape as a term that describes all levels of sexual violence. Stereotypes about what rape involves tend to portray rape as one specific kind of attack. In the law, too, rape is very narrowly defined. But if one defines rape as an assault against someone using sexual behavior as a weapon of domination, rather than as a means of interactive pleasure, then there are a range of 'rapes' in our society.

Research has shown that the trauma involved for women in cases of rape with a foreign object is very much the same as that of rape with a penis. So, too, is the trauma in most other forms of sexual assault, regardless of whether it is between a man and woman, man and man, woman and woman, or adult and child.

It is every person's right to decide with whom they want or do not want to have sex. Even a woman who has invited a man up to her apartment and allows him to kiss, touch and fondle her has the right to say no to sexual intercourse.

Contrary to common belief, rape does not occur because of sexual desire or the need for sexual relief. All men experience sexual desire to a greater or lesser degree, but not all men commit rape. Sexual relief is found by turning to lovers, partners, sex workers or masturbation. Even men with 'healthy' sexual appetites are not necessarily rapists. So why does rape happen?

Rape is an act of power, control, anger, aggression, violence, conquest and degradation aimed at women and expressed through the sexual act. In other words, rapists do not rape for the sake of sexual satisfaction.

Why do men rape?

There are many reasons why men rape.
» They rape for the feeling of power and control that usually accompanies the act of taking someone by force. Generally, the emotions felt by the rapist in this violent act are ones of anger, aggression and frustration, even if only present on a subconscious level.
» They may feel inadequate in one way or another. To counter this feeling of inadequacy and to gain a sense of control, they lash out at women through the act of rape. Here they are in control mentally and physically, and in this way they gain a false sense of power.
» They may rape because they want to prove themselves to their friends and peers. By raping, they achieve a certain amount of status – they 'earn' the right to be included in the group or they gain the 'respect' of the other members. This is especially true in cases of gang rape.
» They may pick up the wrong 'social cue' if a woman is attractive or is nice to them. These men usually have poor relationship and/or social skills.
» They may rape because they do not see women as worthy human beings. Instead, they see women as objects, and their feelings towards women are usually hostile, expecting them to obey without question. These men believe that they can do with women whatever they please, and that 'taking' from women that which has not been given to them freely (sex) is their right.

- » They may rape to release feelings of frustration and anger that they feel either towards women or towards other people and life in general. The women they rape are not necessarily the people with whom they are angry or frustrated.
- » They may rape because they hate and despise women. Rape is a way for them to express this hatred.
- » In certain countries where dowries are still paid by men to the families of their would-be wives, wives are regarded as possessions because they have been 'bought'. These men believe that they are entitled to have sex with their wives whenever they want to, regardless of how their wives feel. If their wives do not comply, are sick, or are not in the mood, the husbands will often rape them anyway.
- » Times of war can also mean that women are more unsafe than usual. It has not been uncommon for invading armies to ravage the land and rape their enemies' women as the ultimate defilement and insult. In this way they are able to assert their authority and power over the men in the communities being invaded. In cultures where dowries have been paid, this is tantamount to theft – they are taking something that does not belong to them, something that other men have paid for. These are definite acts of power and control.

There are some things, however, that are common to all rapists. They have no respect for women and do not see them as worthy beings. Because of this lack of respect, women are obvious targets for the outpouring of anger, aggression, frustration, contempt and abuse.

Lastly, the fact that rape is not about sex but about anger and power is reflected in a statement made by one rapist when he was interviewed: 'I had to get it over with and it was a scary feeling within myself. I had to finish it, I had to hurry up and get away from it. And having sex itself wasn't very enjoyable. But it seemed like a relief for what I was feeling, a way out of my anger inside; a way out was to give it to somebody else and then run, to leave them.'

Who rapes?

All men are capable of committing rape, but most choose not to. The rapist could be a doctor, schoolteacher, mechanic, banker, gardener, accountant, politician, company director, the man next door, an uncle, a boss, a minister of the church, a married man with children – absolutely anyone. There has even been a case where a man confined to a wheelchair lifted a three-year-old girl onto his lap and raped her!

It is not necessarily the stranger who is the rapist, either. Take the example of sexual intercourse between a father and daughter. Despite its technical classification as 'incest', the father uses his position of authority to manipulate and intimidate his daughter for his own pleasure or personal agenda. This is still rape. So is male-on-male, female-on-female, and even the far less common female-on-male forced sexual activity. If anyone is taken in a sexual manner against their will or without their consent, regardless of who it is, that is an act of rape.

> **DID YOU KNOW ...**
>
> » The most common places where rape occurs are in the woman's place of residence, the rapist's place of residence, the rapist's car, and in open spaces (fields, parking lots, parks, sports fields, streets).
> » There is a higher incidence of rape on weekends.
> » More rapes are committed by someone the woman knows or has seen before than by a total stranger.

Social conditioning

To fully understand why rape happens, one must first examine the society we live in and the different social rules we have been expected to follow as men and women. These rules have been ingrained from a very early age, so much so that we are hardly aware of all the little ways in which we conform to them, consciously and unconsciously, day after day.

Schools, churches, recreational activities and even our own homes have been geared, from day one, to establish and reinforce specific roles of behavior for boys and girls.

From the time that a baby is born, his or her conditioning starts. Baby boys have trains, cars, merry-go-rounds, bats and balls painted on their bedroom walls (strong and active). Baby girls have lambs, clouds, rainbows, fairies and teddy bears on theirs (soft and passive). Boys are dressed in blue or green while girls are dressed in pink or yellow. Boys are taught to be aggressors – strong, brave and active, and emotional response is discouraged: 'boys don't cry'. They are also taught to take a stand, because giving in or compromising is seen as a weakness. Girls are encouraged to be passive, well-mannered, quiet, helpful and controlled. Active or assertive response is discouraged: 'little girls don't do that'.

These are all superficial standards that have absolutely nothing to do with what girls and boys are really capable of. Neither do they make any sense. Some typical examples of the effects certain differences in upbringing have on the social and physical skills of boys and girls can be seen in the following table.

EMOTIONAL AND PHYSICAL DIFFERENCES IN BOYS AND GIRLS THROUGH DIFFERENT SOCIAL VALUES	
BOYS	GIRLS
Receive ample physical exercise which enhances strength, co-ordination and muscular structure (climbing trees, running, playing sport, play fighting). This develops confidence in their physical abilities.	Do not receive enough physical exercise with the result that they have less strength and often under-developed muscle structure (are told to climb down from the tree, to stop running around or are not motivated to play sport), and therefore have little confidence in their physical abilities.

EMOTIONAL AND PHYSICAL DIFFERENCES IN BOYS AND GIRLS THROUGH DIFFERENT SOCIAL VALUES	
BOYS	**GIRLS**
Engage in medium to rough contact, enhancing their ability to defend themselves and to withstand medium to heavy blows (play fights, rough-and-tumbles, real fights, or a sport such as rugby).	Receive very little physical contact, resulting in an inability to successfully deal with, and recover from, contact situations (are told to stop fighting and to 'act like ladies', are not encouraged to do semi-contact sports as karate).
Are given toys that promote physical capabilities, for example a ball (to kick), a bat (to hit), a helmet (to protect head in order to play freely), and so on.	Are given toys that promote non-physical capabilities, for example a doll (to nurture and love), a tea set (to serve), a toy telephone (to communicate), and so on.
Are allowed to shout, express themselves, ask for things, stand up for themselves.	Are instructed to be polite, lower their voices and to do as they are told. They are afraid to express themselves assertively.
Are often 'waited on' by their mothers or sisters. They grow up expecting to get what they want from other women.	Perform their own, as well as general, household chores. They grow up believing that their needs and rights are secondary.
Are given tacit authority in the household by being the 'man' of the house and often the one to look after mum when dad is away.	Are given very little or no authority in the household.
Are not allowed to cry and are perceived as 'strong'.	Are allowed to cry and are therefore perceived as 'weak'.
Are expected to be emotionally and physically tough.	Are perceived to be emotionally and physically weak, therefore any so-called weakness is tolerated, even expected.

EMOTIONAL AND PHYSICAL DIFFERENCES IN BOYS AND GIRLS THROUGH DIFFERENT SOCIAL VALUES	
BOYS	GIRLS
Are unduly focused on sex and 'scoring' – they often receive misguided information about sex and love from their peers.	Focus more on love and intimacy than on sex – they are more romantic and idealistic.

By encouraging these differences in children, we are undermining the one (girl) and promoting the other (boy). We are also creating the additional problem of making the girl physically weak and the boy physically strong. This places unrealistic expectations on the boy in that he is expected to be emotionally strong as well – he's not allowed to cry or be afraid of the dark, etc. He comes to believe that this is how a man should be and is often confused by these expectations. The little girl grows into a woman believing that she is physically incompetent and too emotional. She often ignores her very valuable powers of intuition because she is frequently told that she is being over-sensitive and irrational.

Clarissa Pinkola Estés, in her award-winning book *Women who run with the wolves*, explains how girls, usually before the age of five, are taught not to 'see' but to 'make pretty' and 'be nice'. By 'see', Clarissa means 'to see things as they really are'. Girls are encouraged to be polite, keep the peace, be reasonable, make things better, and so on. They are protected from the harsh realities of life and so grow up having idealistic (and often unrealistic) views about love, relationships, life, work and especially men. This makes them naïve.

This early training causes women to override their intuition and encourages them to act in a manner contrary to their deepest convictions. In doing so, they are submitting to the 'predator' and making themselves vulnerable. This becomes particularly relevant when we look at why many women are the victims of rape and assault – naïvety is their greatest enemy. As a result of being naïve, women have lost the ability to differentiate. Differentiation in a self-defence context means being able to tell the difference between the person who is a threat and the one who isn't. Your potential attacker may look 'nice', but you must have the ability to see him for what he really is.

Not only has society made 'victims' of women on an emotional level, but it has disempowered them on a physical level, too. It is no wonder that physical defence is the last thing many women would consider using in a life-threatening situation. They would sooner talk and negotiate their way out of a situation than fight. This is not to say that talking and negotiating are bad, but in a life-threatening situation there inevitably comes a time when one must simply ACT. In other words, when the situation has moved beyond talking and negotiating. Women must learn to identify this turning point and have the confidence to ACT on their convictions.

Developing strength and confidence

In order to change the way men and women relate to and interact with each other, we need to look at changing the way we raise our children. We want children to develop strong character and to have confidence in their own capabilities. To achieve this, we need to allow them to make their own decisions (within reason) about what they like, how they want to play, and with which toys they want to play. We should not force our beliefs and expectations on them – after all, our way is not necessarily their way. Perhaps our sons do not want to be heroes. Maybe our daughters would rather wear blue and climb trees. At this point I would like to emphasize that there is nothing wrong with a girl liking pink and a boy being an ardent sportsman, provided they are choices that have been made without undue influence of family or peers. Instead of sending our children up a one-way street, why not give them a two-way street with an option to go either way?

Changing our focus

Personally, I feel that people should focus on a child's talents – if boys show a talent for the piano or ballet, things you would normally associate with girls, those talents should be developed. The same is true for girls. If they show a talent for carpentry, sport or any other traditionally male-associated activity, these talents should be encouraged.

If you develop children's talents, you will help them build strong character and greater confidence within themselves because they feel good about what they are doing. This creates a feeling of self-worth. Feelings of confidence and self-worth, in turn, provide a sense of internal security and appreciation and respect for other people and their talents. These children will be able to express themselves freely and fully, which contributes to good human relationships between boys and girls, men and women. They will also feel appreciated for what and who they are rather than what or who they should be.

I understand that parents feel concerned when their children climb trees as they could fall and incur injuries. This has an additional set of complications – medical bills, getting them to hospital, taking time off work to look after them, and so on.

We should understand, however, that moving our bodies (kicking a ball, playing in a river, jumping over stones and even climbing a tree) is an essential part of self-discovery – we are discovering things about our own strength, balance, co-ordination and capabilities. Learning to make an effort in doing these things teaches us the value of effort when facing other challenges in life, too.

When a parent says to a girl: 'Don't pick up that chair, let your brother do it,' they are planting a little seed that is saying 'You are weak – your brother is strong. You are not capable, but your brother is,' even if that is not what they mean. What they could say is: 'Please bring me that chair,' and then see how she responds. Let her decide whether she can lift it or not, or, at the very least, give her the opportunity to try – don't simply assume that she can't do it.

A really good example of how society perceives women and how women readily accept these perceptions is reflected in an incident that happened in one of the karate classes I was instructing. My students had to do a series of push-ups. One of my female students got down on the floor and started doing her push-ups from her knees. Puzzled, I asked if she had a back injury. 'No,' she said, and went on to explain: her male gym instructor had asked her to do some push-ups at her last gym but to do them with her knees on the ground. The reason, he said, was because women can't do push-ups!

Instead of encouraging her to do them properly and suggesting that she only do as many as she can manage, he immediately instructed her to do push-ups that were physically less taxing. He never gave her the opportunity to explore her own capabilities. Furthermore, because his position as an instructor implied knowledge and authority, my new student readily accepted his judgement. His attempt to 'accommodate' her would only have weakened and disempowered her in the long run. Incidentally, all the women in my karate classes have successfully managed to do push-ups the proper way!

Overcoming our own limiting perceptions

An interesting example of how our own perceptions can sometimes serve to limit us is illustrated in the following true story:

I used to have a very large whiteboard in my office at home. One day, I single-handedly took it down and placed it up against the wall with the intention of moving it into one of my other rooms. However, because I was running late for an appointment, I asked a friend who was staying with me to move the board when she had a spare moment. Later that afternoon I arrived home to find the board still there.

'Did you forget to move the board?' I asked.

'No,' she said, 'I didn't forget … the board is too heavy.'

'Did you lift the board?' I enquired.

'No,' she replied again, 'it looked too heavy, so I didn't bother.'

Laughing, I told her to give it a try. She did, and lifted it with great ease (whiteboards look a lot heavier than they really are). Needless to say, she felt very embarrassed. It's amazing how limiting your own perceptions can be.

These limiting perceptions can also affect our success in a self-defence situation. Many women automatically assume that their attackers are experienced fighters, that they have attacked many times before and that they are incredibly strong and efficient. These women also perceive themselves to be weak and incapable by comparison.

While I am not advocating that women just blindly and thoughtlessly launch themselves into a self-defence response, I am suggesting that they first assess the situation as objectively as possible, and that they examine their own perceptions in order to determine whether they hold any validity or not, before being too willing to allow them to get in the way.

INTERESTING FACTS

- » 90% of attacks on women are aimed at the upper body first, especially the face and throat area.
- » There are more attacks on women without the use of weapons than there are with weapons.
- » Surveys conducted overseas have indicated that most women who have fought back have successfully prevented an attack. Research has also shown that women who use stronger physical resistance are more likely to avoid rape than women who use less resisitance. Those who do not resist at all are the most likely to be raped, to spend the night in the hospital, and to be robbed.
- » It has been found that women are more likely to use physical resistance against someone who is known to them than against a stranger.
- » Research conducted in America has indicated that vaginal intercourse is the most frequently practiced sexual act in rape (94%), with fellatio being the second highest (17%).

2
PATTERNS OF RAPE

The rapist

It is not possible to point out a would-be rapist. You cannot pick him out in a crowd. He is your everyday man. He looks like other men. Physical attributes, dress and occupation offer no clues to this dark side of his nature. All men can rape, most men choose not to. An interesting point, however, is that when a man does rape, it means that he has either thought about rape, or he has fantasized about it.

Just as there are different motivations for a rape attack, so there are different patterns of attack, and these tend to be closely related. Regardless of which rape pattern is being executed, there are also two basic styles of attack within each pattern, namely the **confidence style** and the **blitz style.**

It is very useful to understand these different patterns and styles, in particular the rape pattern and style with which you are faced. In this way you can more accurately determine your self-defence response.

Keep in mind that one style of attack can easily cross over to the next. In other words, a confidence style of attack could suddenly turn into a blitz style. In certain instances, there can even be a cross-sectioning of patterns – what starts out as date rape could end up as anger rape.

Some rapists tend to stick to one pattern of rape because it is the pattern with which they feel most comfortable and have enacted most often. Other rapists shift between one pattern and the next, either in separate rapes or within a single act of rape.

PATTERNS OF RAPE

The various *patterns* of rape are:
- Confidence rape
- Blitz rape
- Anger rape
- Power rape
- Fantasy rape
- Date rape
- Gang rape
- Convenience rape
- Sadistic rape (organized and disorganized).

CONFIDENCE RAPE

One of the most frequent patterns used by rapists is the confidence pattern. In this pattern, there is an effort to strike up conversation with the person he means to capture. He will try to gain your confidence during this period by means of conversation, anything from a one-minute chat (asking for directions), a three-hour exchange (at a party) or even an exchange over a three-year period (someone with whom you work).

He attempts to gain your confidence throughout his interaction with you. In doing so, you drop your guard, especially when it is someone you have known for a while, or when it is someone that requires your assistance in what appears to be an emergency situation.

This is a difficult pattern to identify as he could be setting you up (he's not attacking you yet). It is also a difficult style of attack to deal with, because this is the pattern where the woman is most likely to engage in internal negotiation, using reason and understanding, and doubting her intuition. After all, he does not appear to be dangerous. Even if there is a seed of doubt in her mind about his intentions, she may still tell herself that she is just being silly. She often thinks: 'What if I'm making a mistake about him?' This is where the naïve woman really gets caught out.

CONFIDENCE RAPE SCENARIOS

1 A young girl is walking home from school. A man pulls up next to her in his car. He looks neat and presentable. He asks her for directions and indicates to her that it would be really helpful if she could show him the way. Needless to say, when she gets into the car she has fallen into his trap.

> **The rapist achieved his goal through communication. He made her feel comfortable and relaxed and made her doubt her own instincts, putting her off-guard.**

Possible response
- » Don't get too close to the car.
- » Don't automatically trust the man talking to you, even if he indicates that he knows your parents or a friend of yours.
- » Tell him that you're sorry, but you can't help him. Don't worry about what he thinks – it doesn't matter if he realizes that you don't trust him. Who is he to you, anyway?
- » Turn away and continue walking away from the car. But stay on guard, he might have another plan of action since his first one failed.

2 A woman works with a male colleague who is married and is the father of two children. They have been working together over a period of three years. One night, while working overtime at the office, he rapes her.

> **He uses his access to her; he uses communication; he gains her confidence over a period of three years so that she feels confident working with him. She thinks that she is safe with him at the office. However, he abuses that trust and rapes her.**

Possible response
- » Even though you know the man, it is important for you to realize that once you are isolated with any man, there is always the possibility of an attack.

- » As he attacks, you must fight back immediately to avoid wasting valuable energy and a good opportunity. Avoid 'negotiating' in your head: 'Why is he doing this to me? He knows me. What have I done wrong?' You should use all of your energy to deal with the attack as effectively as possible. Don't blame yourself.
- » Don't accommodate the man when he attacks you.
- » Although you may have worked for a number of years with a male colleague who is married and has children, it does not mean you are safe and he cannot rape. These assumptions often get women into trouble. Follow your intuition the minute you sense his energy changing towards you. At this early stage, you could still possibly talk your way out of the situation. If that is not possible, you must remember that you have a right to defend yourself physically.

3 A nurse walks along a footpath back to the hostel after her duties. She gets attacked, thrown to the ground, and then raped. Another man comes to her assistance and screams at the man raping her, 'What are you doing?'. The attacker jumps up and runs away. The man that comes to her rescue helps her onto her feet and puts his arm around her. She is distraught and crying, and he says, 'Don't worry, everything will be fine.' He offers to take her to the police station. She trusts him, and he has gained her confidence because she needs his help. He suddenly throws her to the ground and rapes her.

> He has gained her trust by coming to her assistance and assuring her that everything will be alright. He has taken advantage of her vulnerable emotional and mental state.

Possible response

This is a difficult situation as the average woman would genuinely believe that she is going to be helped. This is an example of the lengths to which a rapist using the confidence pattern will actually go. Be on guard at all times and never take anything for granted. If in any way possible, keep your mind strong and be prepared to fight back.

4 A woman is standing outside a lift. The doors open and an ordinary-looking man wearing a suit and holding a briefcase says: 'Are you going up or down?' She says, 'I'm going down,' and gets into the lift. He pushes the basement button, then he grabs her around the throat and pushes her against the side of the lift. He takes her down to the basement, drags her out and rapes her.

> Within a couple of seconds, through simple communication that appears to be friendly and helpful, he catches her off-guard.

Possible response
- » The first thing you must ask yourself as the door opens is: 'Do I feel comfortable with this person?' (what is your intuition telling you?).
- » If you feel uncomfortable, don't get into the lift. Rather say: 'It's okay, you go – I am waiting for a friend.'
- » If you do get into the lift, make sure you're standing near the buttons. If you realize you've made a mistake, immediately push the buttons of all floors, and get out as quickly as possible. The lift doors will open on every floor, making it difficult for your attacker to continue.

BLITZ RAPE

Blitz rape is when you are attacked out-of-the-blue. In other words, you do not see it coming. Most blitz attacks happen from behind or from the side.

The blitz attacker is not interested in communicating with you – as a matter of fact, if you try to talk to him, you might only end up irritating him, thereby running the risk of spoiling your good chances to fight back. If you scream for help, he could kill you immediately. The attack is hard and fast. The attacker could strike at you, tear your clothes, push, grab, slap, or even jump on top of you. His presence is inappropriate, he is uninvited and he forces himself into the situation. The blitz attacker also tends to be a stranger, someone you have never seen before.

BLITZ RAPE SCENARIOS

1 A woman is in her office one night, listening to the radio and finishing off some work. Suddenly somebody grabs her around the throat from behind and holds a screwdriver to her neck.

> Her attacker has sneaked up on her and taken her by surprise. Her radio has masked any noise that she might otherwise have heard. Her attacker does not speak to her, but gets straight down to business by launching into his attack.

Possible response
- » It is highly unlikely that talking to or attempting to reason with this man will achieve anything.
- » If you are sure there are people nearby, you can try screaming loudly. This could scare him off.
- » Identify his vulnerable body target areas (see pages 68–70) and apply the appropriate self-defence techniques to those areas as quickly and as hard as possible.
- » Run away at the earliest opportunity.

2 A woman is out jogging in her neighbourhood. Suddenly a man jumps out and attacks her from the side, grabs her around her arms and body, drags her off the path to a nearby bush, and throws her to the ground.

> This attack seems to come from nowhere. As with the first blitz scenario, there is no communication between the attacker and the victim, and there are no preliminaries. This type of attack is hard, fast, and without warning.

Possible response
- » If thrown to the ground, try to get up as quickly as possible unless you are familiar with, and proficient in, self-defence ground techniques. Should you be thrown onto loose sand, grab a handful and throw it into your attacker's face and eyes. This will give you time to get up and fight back and/or run away.
- » The response from Blitz Rape Scenario 1 would be applicable in this situation.

ANGER RAPE

The anger rapist uses sexual assault to express his anger and rage towards women or, more specifically, a woman in his life that has upset, hurt or angered him. The woman he rapes is not necessarily the person that has triggered this response. In fact, any upsetting incident – losing a job, being reprimanded or humiliated – could trigger this reaction, which is then taken out on women because the anger rapist has little or no regard for them.

Anger rape is executed in an explosive manner: the attack is normally aggressive and the impact is hard. The rapist often uses more force than is necessary to control his victim. The underlying feelings of intense anger, frustration and discontent are apparent. This style of rape seems to be more impulsive than premeditated. The rapist could also swear at his victim, spit on her, use extremely foul and offensive language and make her submit to additional degrading acts. It is very important for the woman not to take this personally.

ANGER RAPE SCENARIOS

1 A man has an argument with his girlfriend. Feeling immediate and extreme anger, he storms out of the house. He spots a woman standing at the bus stop. His intense anger prompts him to initiate an attack on this woman and to rape her.

> **The rapist initiates a spontaneous attack and rapes the woman in an effort to give vent to his rage and anger. His whole attitude is aggressive, angry, hostile and violent.**

Possible response
» It is highly unlikely that talking to or attempting to reason with this man will achieve anything.

» The rapist is angry and will probably use more force than is necessary to overpower and rape you. Your response should be very strong, using techniques on target – there is little room for error because it's either him or you. Decide, without question, that it's going to be him.
» Identify his vulnerable body target areas and apply appropriate techniques to those areas as quickly and as hard as possible.
» Screaming could further anger him and should probably only be used if he attacks you in an area that is more exposed, with people nearby.
» Get away at the earliest opportunity.

2 A teenage boy is reprimanded and belittled by a female teacher in front of the other students. Embarrassed and angry, he stands up and storms out. A few blocks away from the school he comes across a girl and, still angry at the teacher, rapes her.

> **The teenage boy feels humiliated and belittled. He probably harbours other unresolved issues such as feelings of anger and resentment towards women in general or a female family member in particular. His teacher's behavior triggers these unresolved feelings and he experiences immediate anger which he takes out on an innocent girl.**

Possible response
» The same as Anger Rape Scenario 1.

POWER RAPE

With power rape, the attacker usually uses only whatever force is required to overpower his victim. He uses verbal threats and often intimidates the victim with a weapon. His motives for raping are often a lack of power or sense of inadequacy that he feels within himself. Raping provides him with the sense of power, strength and control that he feels he lacks.

POWER RAPE SCENARIOS

1. A man accosts a woman in a parking garage, pushes her into his car and threatens to hurt her if she does not co-operate. He rapes her. He talks to her briefly and has a cigarette. He then drags her to an unused stairwell, again threatening to hurt her if she does not comply. He rapes her again.

> The rapist uses the threat of violence to force the woman to co-operate. This threat can be either a manipulative tactic or real. He uses whatever force is necessary to achieve his objectives.

Possible response
» Take a good look at your attacker: he may not be adequate. The fact that he has to use threats to control and manipulate you suggests that he may not be as competent as he would like you to think he is. Good, strong, focused techniques on your part will be very effective.

2. A man holds a knife to a woman's throat as she's about to enter her house. He instructs her to do as he says or he'll use the knife. He takes her inside and rapes her. While he's raping her he asks if she's enjoying it, if this is the best she's ever had. Scared, she says 'I don't know'. He becomes angry and says, 'Tell me! Is this the best you've ever had?' Afraid, she says 'Yes, it's the best'. Satisfied with this, he finishes raping her, ties her up and leaves.

> The rapist used only the force necessary to gain co-operation. He needs affirmation of his potency and manhood, even if it is forced. It never occurs to him that what he is doing is wrong. He wants to believe that she means it when she says he's the best.

Possible response
» Same as Power Rape Scenario 1.

FANTASY RAPE

The fantasy rape pattern involves the rapist fantasizing about the rape before he actually does it. The victim could be a woman he has fantasized about in particular, or someone that conveniently fits into a fantasy he has already created in his mind (she may look the same as his fantasy woman). He is possibly one of the few rapists who will watch and follow you over a period of anything from a few weeks to a few months. He will often monitor his potential victim's movements and routine in order to plan his attack. This is part of his thrill. He also uses this time to build his fantasy.

The rapist will go to extreme lengths to get to his potential victim: He is quite prepared to climb up a drainpipe to access a woman's apartment located on the fifth floor. He will break through burglar bars to get into her bedroom, rape her and then, strangely enough, exit through her front door.

He normally enters the woman's apartment when she is sleeping. Many women have woken to find a man standing in their bedroom, watching or staring at them, or have felt a heavy weight pouncing on them.

The fantasy rapist sometimes apologizes to his victim after the rape. He may also threaten her by saying that he will come back and do it again if she calls the police. However, he rarely does.

It's not uncommon for this rapist to lose his erection halfway through the rape, as he realizes that it is not living up to his fantasy. This, in turn, makes him feel inadequate and so he will try again with someone else, thinking, 'next time it will be better'. The loss of his erection normally signals the end of his current attempt.

FANTASY RAPE SCENARIOS

1 A woman wakes up to find a man standing naked next to her bed. He tells her that she's so beautiful, he's been watching her, and he knows that they'd be wonderful together. When she starts screaming he gets upset and angry. Immediately he covers her mouth and tells her that he doesn't

want to hurt her ... he just wants to love her. She starts struggling and he jumps on top of her, telling her that it doesn't have to be this way. Pulling off her nightclothes, he rapes her. When he has finished he gets up and puts his clothes back on. He apologizes to her, and warns her not to contact the police or he'll come back to get her. After this, he leaves quietly.

> The rapist has built up a fantasy about this woman and truly believes that she will want and desire him when he presents himself to her. He apologizes to her afterwards, not because he genuinely regrets what he has done, but because he is sorry it had to be done that way.

Possible response
» He is naked, making his whole body a wonderful target area. Not only can you clearly see the target areas, but there is no clothing to protect them. Stay calm, identify these target areas (groin first because, from a lying or sitting position, it is the most accessible), then apply your self-defence techniques hard onto the identified area. Follow up this technique with another technique, and another, until he either tries to get away or you have managed to immobilize him. Remove yourself from the apartment immediately. Run to a neighbour and telephone the police.

2 A female student in a room on the third floor of a college residence wakes up to find a man standing alongside her bed. Shocked, but in control, she asks him how on earth he managed to get into her room. Rather proud of himself, he tells her how, for weeks, he has been studying the building and his planned route to her room. 'But it's three stories high!' she exclaims. 'How did you do it?' The potential rapist leads her to the window and, pointing outside, shows her the exact route he has taken to her room.

> The rapist has clearly stated that he has studied and planned his entry into her room for the past few weeks. True to the fantasy rapist pattern, he enters the room while she is asleep.

Possible response

» Engaging in conversation (centred around the rapist's entry to the room) has bought this girl a few extra minutes of time. It has served to put the rapist off-guard and given the girl a chance to compose herself and think of an action plan.
» She could execute a strike or kick to any of the rapist's target areas, and then follow that up with other self-defence techniques until he is immobilized.
» She should remove herself from the room immediately and call for help.

DATE RAPE

The date rapist uses the date as an opportunity to get close to you without evoking any suspicion. He puts you in a setting that is both comfortable and convenient for him to rape you. He does not necessarily rape you on the first date, but if he follows the date rape pattern, it is likely that he will rape you on the third or fourth date.

In the book *Why Men Rape* by Sylvia Levine and Joseph Koenig, a rape offender says: 'All of my rapes have been in a dating situation where I've been out with woman who I know … I wouldn't take no for an answer. I think it had something to do with my acceptance of rejection. I had low self-esteem and not much self-confidence and when I was rejected for something which I considered to be rightly mine, I became angry and I went ahead anyway.'

DATE RAPE SCENARIOS

1 A woman and her new date arrive back at her apartment after an evening out. He invites himself up to her apartment for coffee. Not sure whether she wants that, she hesitates, then gives in. As soon as they are in the apartment, he grabs her, pushes her up against the wall and starts to remove her clothing. She tries to struggle but he does not release his grip. He calls her a tease, then rapes her.

> The rapist has used the date to gain her confidence and to gain access to a suitable place in which to rape her. He tries to make her feel guilty by telling her that she is a tease (and therefore the rape is her fault).

Possible response
- If you so much as feel the slightest hesitation, DO NOT allow your date to come up to your apartment. Trust your intuition and instincts. Make an excuse if you have to. Say that you're too tired, you want to go straight to bed and perhaps you'll have coffee another time. If he makes you feel uncomfortable, try to avoid being alone with him. Better still, always try to find your own way home after a new date. Call a friend to pick you up if you don't have a car, or call a taxi.
- No matter what he says, he has NO right to rape you. Not even if you've allowed him to kiss and fondle you. Every person has a right to draw their limits.
- Otherwise, any close-range self-defence techniques will be suitable. Execute them as accurately and with as much power as possible.

GANG RAPE

This pattern involves group participation in the rape. The gang sees the victim purely as an object. What often happens is that the leader takes the initiative and, by his example, encourages the rest of the group to follow. Often this type of rape is used to establish individual status within the group. Their behavior is violent and it dehumanizes the victim. There has, however, been a case of a woman getting out of a gang rape situation by 'playing up to' the leader and suggesting that she wants him first. By getting him to one side, away from the group, she had an opportunity to talk to him. She told him that he seemed different from the rest, that he looked like a really nice guy. She tried to get him to see that he had nothing to prove and appeared to be the type of person that could be reasonable. When the others in the group demanded their turn, the leader refused and he protected her from them. This is not to say that I recommend the same course of action to other women in this situation, but simply that, in this instance, the woman's instincts on how to handle the situation paid off.

GANG RAPE SCENARIO

1 A woman is walking along the road when a car stops and a man gets out. He grabs her and pulls her into the car. There are three other men already there. They take her to a nearby forest, drag her out of the car, tie her hands to a tree and rape her, one by one. When they have finished, they drive away, leaving her still tied to the tree.

> The rape is more about the gang than about the woman. They could be bored and out looking for a little 'sport'. They could also be trying to prove something to each other.

Possible response
» If there were only two men and she was quite proficient at self-defence, she would have a good chance of getting out of the situation – the techniques she uses on the one could be used on the other. An effective technique is an effective technique.
» It is very difficult to suggest a course of action where there are more than two rapists. The woman has to rely entirely on her intuition and what her instincts are telling her to do.
» Women who go to nightclubs must be specially cautioned: be aware and very careful that your drinks have not been spiked (had drugs added to them). This is a popular ploy by rapists, including gang rapists. Do not allow yourself to be led outside alone by any man. It is very easy to get raped that way. Watch your drinks at all times and do not accept a drink from anyone unless you have actually seen it being poured.

CONVENIENCE RAPE

Convenience rape is seldom premeditated. The primary motivation would normally be a burglary or some other unrelated activity.

    A good example of this pattern is where the attacker's main intention is the burglary of a woman's house and the woman happens to arrive home, rather conveniently for the attacker. He decides to rape her while he's there. Or, a man breaks into a house with the intent of stealing, walks into the bedroom, finds a woman sleeping, and decides to rape her.

CONVENIENCE RAPE SCENARIOS

1 A man enters a house in the early hours of the morning. He starts stuffing CDs into a pillowcase he has found. He then moves into the next room, only to find a woman there, sleeping. The rapist wakes her and, threatening her with a knife, asks her for all her money. Seeing her in a nightshirt, he decides he'd like a bit of fun, and orders her to undress. Scared of the knife, she does. He rapes her.

> The rapist entered the house with the primary intention of stealing. He had not specifically planned to rape. A suitable victim happened to be there and he thought he'd take advantage of the opportunity.

Possible response
- While she should not take the weapon (knife) lightly, she should also not empower the rapist so readily. He may simply carry it to assist him with his burglaries should he find himself confronted unexpectedly.
- Look for an opportunity to implement your self-defence techniques. Remember, there are different stages in an attack, and any one of these stages could provide you with a suitable opening.
- You could tell him that he doesn't need the knife because you will co-operate with him. Casually suggest that he put down the knife because you will give him what he wants. If he puts it down, take advantage of the

opportunity and apply your self-defence techniques. But move quickly! Get to him before he can retrieve the knife.

SADISTIC RAPE (ORGANIZED AND DISORGANIZED)

In a sadistic rape pattern the attacker often uses an instrument or foreign object such as a bottle, stick or screwdriver with which to rape his victim. His attack is brutal and of a sadistic nature – he gets high on attacking his victim in this way. He could tie her to the bed or a tree, cut off her breast, rape her, cut off the other breast and rape her again. He finds gratification in hurting, degrading, controlling and destroying his victim. He could show an abnormal tendency such as an anti-social disorder or schizophrenia. Very often the sadistic rapist will kill his victim. There are two kinds of sadistic rapist: the **organized rapist** and the **disorganized rapist**.

The organized sadistic rapist is usually a man with a high IQ who is neatly dressed and healthy looking. He likes to exercise, drives a clean car and lives in a clean apartment/house. He has an impressive personality (charming) and speaks with confidence. Often he has a 'rape kit' in his car and his rapes are premeditated. The rape kit could include tape, handcuffs, rope, a knife, scissors, gloves, a balaclava, and so on. Because of his charming manner, the organized sadistic rapist will often use the confidence style of attack in an attempt to establish some form of communication with you first. In this way, he can more easily lure you into his trap.

The disorganized sadistic rapist looks unclean, unkempt, unhealthy and cannot hold a job long. He lives in an unclean place and if he drives a car, the car will be unclean or even damaged on the outside. His attacks are not premeditated, neither are they well planned – if he enters your house and attacks you, he will not necessarily have a getaway car. This is the perfect example of his 'disorganized mind'. (He won't think about fingerprints either.) He tends to use the blitz style of attack, although he could use the confidence style, too. The confidence style of attack, however, would almost certainly lead into a blitz attack.

STYLES OF ATTACK

Confidence style

This is when your attacker communicates with you in order to gain your confidence and to get you off-guard. Once he has achieved this, his style of attack changes to the blitz style, where he moves in and attacks you without warning. When the confidence style of attack is in progress, you can play for time by talking to your potential attacker, keeping him at a distance and redirecting his attention. While you are talking to him and your senses are telling you that this is a potential attacker, you can think of a plan of action to get away, even before he attacks you. For instance, you can remove yourself from the situation altogether by saying, 'Sorry, I can't help you', and then immediately walk away.

Blitz style

This is when the rapist attacks you out-of-the-blue. There is no warning and it happens very quickly. The blitz attacker seldom communicates with you – if he was interested in talking he would have followed the confidence style of attack.

In the blitz attack, your attacker has already leapt out of his starting blocks – there is nothing left for you to do but implement your self-defence with determination and purpose.

The impact of the attack is normally hard, aggressive and forceful.

3
DYNAMICS OF SELF-DEFENCE

On average, only 10% of women forcefully resist when being raped.

Women often fear for their lives, and understandably so, because what may start out as a simple burglary could easily change into a violent situation resulting in the woman being tied up and raped, even killed.

The application of self-defence techniques should be highly favoured as an option that would be not only effective, but that would also surprise your attacker.

A survey conducted in America showed that women who took on a firmer or more aggressive stance during an attack were the ones that were more likely to get out of their attack situations.

During 1990, of one thousand women examined after being raped in the Gauteng area, only 10% showed signs of resistance, mostly in the form of pushing the attacker back or covering their faces. There were no indications that self-defence techniques had been used. The other 90% had not resisted at all. It must also be understood that there is a big difference between resisting/struggling and the application of effective self-defence techniques.

It is not that the average woman cannot defend herself, but rather that she does not know *how* to defend herself. The appropriate responses to the different attack situations featured in this book have been specially selected with the 'average' women in mind. In other words, no particular level of physical fitness or previous experience in self-defence is required to be able to implement, or benefit from, the techniques illustrated here. However, a certain level of physical fitness does contribute towards success in your counter-action since there are no guarantees as to how long an attack might last. One minute of fighting can feel like thirty minutes – your adrenalin is pumping, your heart rate goes up and a tremendous amount of energy is expended.

Remember, should you find yourself in a situation where you must defend yourself, stay calm and stay supple. By staying calm your thinking processes will be far clearer and you will be able to make better decisions about how to deal with the attack. If you are hysterical, you will struggle to handle the situation effectively, both emotionally and physically. You will also tire yourself very quickly. By staying supple, your body will be able to generate energy through easier movement, which in turn will support your self-defence techniques.

Moving your body is a method of defence that makes you less available to your attacker – it is harder for him to grab you and attack you. It is also easier for you to take off quickly after you have applied your techniques (attack/counter-attack). In other words, body movement is used for both defence and attack/counter-attack.

In order to be successful in self-defence you have to:
» make a mind shift
» develop mental strength
» develop emotional strength/stability
» develop physical ability
» have commitment
» maintain endurance.

ATTITUDE comes first ... self-defence, second.

The mind shift

I cannot stress strongly enough how important the correct mind shift is in any confrontational situation. In most cases, your frame of mind or attitude during an attack will determine whether or not you are successful in warding off your attacker.

It is very important to have a true and urgent desire to get out of your situation; a willingness to do whatever it takes to achieve that desire; determination; strong attitude; and a knowledge of basic, effective self-defence techniques applied with as much power as you can physically muster onto the vulnerable target areas of your attacker's body.

Adopting the right frame of mind involves making a complete mind shift from your old way of thinking to a new, powerful, more positive way of thinking that will empower you and motivate you into action.

Creating a mind shift could also mean doing things you would never normally do, such as spitting into your attacker's face or poking his eyes.

Connecting mind and body

To understand the importance of the mind in self-defence, you must first understand how the mind works.

Very briefly, when you want to spring into action, your brain sends messages to various muscles in your body telling them *when* and *how* to perform the necessary movements. These messages govern how quickly your muscles respond and how strong or fast your techniques are. If your mind is confused and you do not know what to do, the correct messages will not get through to your muscles. Your body will react accordingly – it becomes confused and uncoordinated, and any techniques you perform will end up being 'wishy-washy' and ineffective.

For this reason, it is imperative that you try to think as clearly as possible and avoid panic. In a defence situation, your attacker is your first enemy, panic your second. Panic confuses, immobilizes and reduces the focus necessary for effective defence and escape.

In my experience, women who find themselves in a physically confrontational situation often tend to 'lose it' mentally. They struggle to think clearly and become removed from what is happening to them – a kind of 'mind freeze' – much like the proverbial deer on the road that is immobilized by the approaching headlights of a car.

Your way of thinking is very important throughout the fight. One of the things you must ask yourself is: **Do I really want to get out of this?** If your answer is 'yes', then you must ACT!

It is essential that you keep your thoughts together throughout your fight. Doing this will help to keep your mind uncluttered and enable it to function more neutrally, giving you the ability to recognize opportunities to fight back and escape as and when they arise.

Accepting and internalizing some of the following statements will help you to make the right mind shift:
- » Nobody has the right to hurt me.
- » I have the right to hurt my attacker (my life is at stake or my children's lives are in danger).
- » I'm going to empower myself, *not* the attacker.
- » I have the element of surprise on my side.
- » I am going to take the control and authority away from the attacker.
- » I am in a difficult situation, but I'm going to deal with it.
- » I am a smart, strong, capable woman.
- » I accept that I can get physically hurt, either by him attacking me, or by me attacking him.
- » I am a worthy person.
- » I do not want to be another statistic.
- » I have a storehouse of effective weapons: I can use my hands, fingers, nails, knees, elbows, feet, legs, arms, voice, teeth, head, etc. I can poke his eyes, elbow him, kick him, head-bang him, spit at him, punch him, grab his hair, scratch him, etc.
- » I can see.
- » I can hear.
- » I can throw things at him.
- » I can yell.
- » I can jump over tables or chairs to get away.
- » I can bite*.
- » I can talk.
- » I can pivot my body.

*Because of the risk of AIDS, we recommend this technique as a last resort.

Mental strength

Just as you have to make the appropriate mind shift, adequate mental strength is necessary and should be developed, too:
- » I will maintain a strong attitude throughout my ordeal.

- » I believe I am going to get out of this alive.
- » I will not give up – if I go down, he will go down with me.
- » I have been hurt, but I will not allow my pain to prevent me from fighting back.
- » I am determined.
- » I will trust my instincts.
- » I will stay smart and alert.

Emotional strength and stability

Emotional strength and stability are often a lot easier to achieve once the correct mind shift has been made and the appropriate mental attitude adopted. Some examples of emotional strength and stability are:

- » I must empower myself.
- » He's slapped my face and thrown me hard onto the ground. Am I going to lie there like a bag of potatoes or am I going to get up and deal with this situation? (This is the emotional trigger needed to pick yourself up off the ground.) I must be emotionally strong, pick myself up and carry on. I must not allow my feelings of fear, pain or self-pity to immobilize me or make me weak. I must empower myself.
- » He is swearing at me. I will switch off emotionally to this abuse. I won't take what he says personally. I will hold my resolve. I will not compromise myself or allow myself to become paralyzed by his insults. What does it matter what he thinks or feels? I will not allow him to disarm me emotionally with something that is of no importance. I must empower myself.

Physical ability

The next step is to develop physical competence:

- » Develop the physical ability to execute self-defence techniques – body movement, stamina/fitness, power, speed, point of focus, timing, agility, co-ordination, balance, muscle strength.
- » Practise your techniques regularly so that they feel more familiar. Regular practice helps to programme the correct muscle response.

These elements will be dealt with in greater depth further on in the book.

Commitment

You should develop commitment to your cause as this is the essential ingredient that will see you through:
- » Follow through with what you have started.
- » Execute your self-defence techniques with both commitment and determination.
- » Have confidence in your ability and decisions.
- » What he has started, you must finish.

Endurance

- » Don't give up.
- » Push your efforts that much further.
- » If plan A doesn't work, try plan B, then plan C, until you are successful.
- » Stay with each moment – avoid the temptation to distance yourself mentally.
- » No matter how tired you are, keep going.
- » Keep believing you will pull through.

YOUR ATTITUDE

The walk

Often women look like 'walking victims', unsure of themselves, shy and naïve. Walk with confidence. Your walk should indicate that you know exactly where you are going, even if you don't. Avoid listening to music or podcasts through earphones while walking. While this may help to pass the time, it distracts you from what is happening around you and it will be difficult to hear a potential attacker approaching. From an attacker's perspective, your lack of awareness makes you an easy target. Walk with your head up so that your surroundings are visible to you and you are aware of what's happening around you. Generate strong, positive energy while you are walking.

The look

When you open your front door, look at the person standing in front of you and project an attitude of confidence. Your tone of voice should generate a feeling of being sure of yourself. Do not let the person know that you are alone.

Very often, an attacker will play on your feelings of sympathy or try to gain your trust in order to get inside your home. For instance, he may say that his car has broken down and he needs to use your phone to call for help. Simply tell him that your phone is not working and/or you've run out of airtime. Or he may say that he has an emergency. Ask what the emergency is and, if you feel compelled to help, offer to call the police, ambulance or locksmith on his behalf. **Do not let him in**. If you have a security gate, it should be **kept locked at all times**. If you do not have one, remember to immediately close and lock the door *before* turning away from him. It is also advisable to keep your conversation to a minimum. Remember, if he is an attacker looking for an opportunity, he is using the 'confidence style' and he will keep trying to gain your trust by engaging you in conversation until he eventually wins you over and you let him in.

If you have an uneasy feeling about him, phone your Neighbourhood Watch immediately. Avoid opening the door again at all costs. If he does not leave after you've closed the door, he is obviously there to do more than just use the telephone and may move to another access point around the house. Fortunately, backup will already be on its way. If you did not make the call before, NOW is the time to do it!

Remember: even if he is legitimately seeking help, you do not need to help him and you do not need to feel bad for not doing so. A decent man will understand why, and will have no problem seeking help elsewhere.

Your space

Always be aware of the space around you, and especially of anyone entering that space. If you have realized that someone is about to attack you, try to have an automatic response the moment he enters that space. In order to identify your space, draw an imaginary circle around you. When your attacker enters that circle, you must react! Remember, he has moved into your space which places you in a position of danger. The fact that he has moved into your space is justification enough for a steadfast and undoubting reaction from your side.

Playing rough

You must be prepared to play rough because your attacker is going to be rough. He could throw you against the wall, onto the floor, or up against a tree. Do not waste valuable energy feeling sorry for yourself. Feeling sorry for yourself is an emotional response that will result in your being soft and ineffective – it will dampen and kill your spirit. Rather channel your energy into planning how to get away. If you can adopt a mental and emotional attitude of, 'How dare he? He has no right to do that!', your fighting spirit will be greatly enhanced and you will find the energy needed to fight back.

Never trust your attacker

Never trust your attacker, even if he pleads with you. This is all part of his pattern, his ploy to catch you out. He is playing on your sensitivities, thinking 'she will feel sorry for me', or 'she will be understanding'. He will take full advantage of your weak moment and will not excuse you for it.

Following through

Be prepared to continue your initial action with an ongoing attack. In other words, do not limit yourself to a one-technique response. Try to follow up on that technique with another technique, and another one, until you have immobilized your attacker, either temporarily or permanently.

If you have succeeded in knocking your attacker to the floor, one of two things are possible:

» You can use a follow-up technique, for example, grabbing something with which you can hit him over the head (with the intention of knocking him unconscious); or

» As he drops down onto the ground you can turn around and run away. Be aware that if you turn your back on him you are exposing yourself to an attack from behind, unless your blow has dazed him for a couple of seconds. If other people are nearby, screaming or shouting for help as you run away will likely deter him from coming after you.

Commitment

Once you take off and execute your first technique, you must have **total commitment**. If you are not committed to what you are doing, you will end up doing it half-heartedly, with the result that your techniques may not be very effective. Be serious about wanting to stop the attack and maintain a strong attitude throughout your fight. Your desire and willingness to get out of your situation alive should be your main motivation and strength.

Determination

Don't give up easily. Your attacker may not be very fit or strong, and he may not have a backup plan, either. This could be his first attack and he may not be experienced, or he may not have expected you to fight back as you are and decides that it's more trouble than it's worth. Endurance on your part is very important and could mean that you manage to outlast and even outwit him.

If plan A doesn't work, move to plan B, then plan C, and so on. Change back to plan A again, if necessary, but DON'T GIVE UP. You are a lot stronger than you think you are. You have internal strength that cannot be anticipated by your attacker – strength that can help you keep going even when your body feels that it physically can't. There are amazing stories of mothers picking up incredible weights to save their children from being crushed or killed, simply because they were desperate to save them.

Intuition/Instinct

Women are born with the wonderful power of intuition. It is the one great asset that we have that men generally don't have or have to work a lot harder to tap into.

We lose this power because, as young girls, we are overprotected and this power is not encouraged. It is also often dismissed by those around us, especially men. Their attitude is: If it cannot be proven or physically seen, it does not exist.

As women, we must seek to redevelop our powers of intuition by placing more trust in what we sense. In other words, we should not dismiss things we have a gut feel about. By using this incredible sense, we might prevent an attack by not walking into a situation we have a bad feeling about.

Fear of failing and taking risks

Generally, women have a great fear of failing and of taking risks. They are inclined to want guarantees before they commit themselves to something.

Women *can* physically hurt men, but most are afraid of doing so. Some women, because they do not have confidence in their own strength, believe that if they hurt men, men will get angry and hurt them back more.

Women also don't like causing damage or hurt to others. Perhaps this is because of their upbringing as nurturers, as the ones who have to look after men.

The nature of women is also that of 'natural peacemaker' as opposed to 'natural fighter'. Keep in mind that you are probably going to get hurt *anyway* during the attack, whether you fight back or not, and that there are no guarantees.

PHYSICAL CONSIDERATIONS

Body movement and proper stances

How you move your body is of utmost importance during an attack. There are many ways in which you can move your body, some of the most obvious being forwards, backwards, to the left and to the right. You can also step, slide, wriggle around, spin, twist, jump, duck, pivot, and so on.

Whenever possible, you should stand firmly upright with your feet shoulder-width apart, your back leg locked straight and your front leg slightly in front (see page 72). This will help you to secure good balance and support for your upper body and will also ensure the proper foundation for your counter-attack.

Your attacker will most probably be bigger than you, therefore your upper body will, in all likelihood, receive the initial blows. This could include a punch to your face, a stranglehold on your neck with one or both of his hands from the front or from behind, pulling your hair, or covering your mouth, to name but a few. Having a good, solid stance will enable you to handle these blows more effectively without you ending up in an even more compromising position, such as on the floor.

The situation may also be such that you have to twist and slide your body from one position to the next (a potentially unstable movement). When you land, however, you should resume a good and solid stance as quickly as possible.

Distance

It is important that you are aware of the distance between you and your attacker. Sometimes you may need to shift your body to successfully apply certain techniques. A punch to the throat or face requires that you are a lot closer to your attacker than, say, a kick to his groin.

Maintaining proper distance is also useful as a preventative measure, for example when someone knocks at your door and you make a move to open it. Don't open the door and take a step forward. You should open it and take a step backwards. This places more distance between you and the potential attacker. This will enable you to see his actions before he actually reaches you. If you have a security gate, be careful not to stand too close to it. The potential attacker can still grab at you through the bars.

My advice to elderly or less agile women is to keep a self-defence spray (mace spray) with you when you open the door. Hold it in the hand that feels most comfortable, ensuring that the nozzle is pointed in the right direction should you have to use it. Then, keeping that hand behind your back, open the door with your other hand, stepping backwards as you do so. Should you need to use the spray, you can simply pull it out and spray, confident that you will be spraying directly into your attacker's face. Trying to grab the spray later on and then fumbling to point it in the right direction will cost you valuable time. Be prepared when you open the door. A few seconds are all that is needed to be overpowered!

Power and speed

Needless to say, it is very important to physically practise all self-defence techniques to ensure proper co-ordination between your mind and your body. Practising these techniques will also help you develop the power and speed necessary for maximum effectiveness.

Techniques should always be applied accurately onto the **target areas** of the attacker's body with as much power and speed as you can manage (see body target areas on pages 68–70). The disadvantage of a slow technique is that your attacker will likely see it coming before it lands, and deflect it. Maintain your sharpness.

If you have space in your home, setting up a punching bag is a great option. You can use it to release daily stress, build up some cardio fitness, and practise punching and kicking with power and speed. Regular exercise using a punching bag will also help you build endurance.

Ground surface

Chances are high that the surface of the ground, as well as the setting, will be neither as safe nor as desirable as you would wish them to be. For example, you could be lying on the beach where the surface is soft sand. You could be sleeping in bed where the surface is the mattress. Or you could be pushed down onto rough, hard tarmac.

NEVER drop down to the ground voluntarily unless you are confident in self-defence ground techniques. If you are knocked down, get up quickly and adopt a solid stance (see page 72). If that is not possible, grab onto any items within your reach for support or that you can use as a weapon in your defence. For example, grab sand and fling it in his eyes if you're on the beach, or push a coffee table into his legs if you're lying on the lounge floor.

The environment

Again, your environment may be less than desirable: it could be raining, making the surface quite slippery; it may be dark, making it difficult to see and identify target areas on the attacker's body; you could be in an enclosed space, making breathing difficult, or in a small or narrow space, making it difficult to move freely.

All these factors could mean that you are not as successful with your techniques. Regardless of your situation, it is important to recover as quickly as possible and try again. Your ongoing fighting spirit may just make him feel that the effort is not worthwhile and result in him giving up. Also keep in mind that your attacker is exposed to the same environmental factors that you are, so if you are experiencing difficulty, so is he!

Stay alert

NEVER take your eyes off your attacker and NEVER underestimate him, not because he is better than you, but to ensure that you are ready and alert at all times. In this way you will give it your best. If you work from the platform that your attacker is powerful and strong, you will apply your techniques with maximum power and strength as well. Watch your attacker because he might change his plan of action. For example, he could suddenly pull out a knife, or he could be hesitating in his attack pattern. As long as you look at him and stay alert, you will have a better chance of seeing what is coming next.

Timing

On a technical level, a good sense of timing can help you deliver self-defence techniques when they are most effective – if you block too early, you are still an open target; if you block too late, your attacker will have made contact.

Remember, the surprise element of your counter-attack is always a positive factor. To maintain the surprise, automatic responses are preferable as these give your attacker very little warning of your intentions.

Good timing also means taking full advantage of brief moments of opportunity to apply your techniques, for instance, the attacker is not focused; he is momentarily distracted; he has taken his eyes off you for a few seconds (to open a car door, to unzip his trousers, or to make sure no one is watching); he is trying to recover from a blow that you may have already delivered, and so on.

One of the questions I frequently hear at my workshops is 'When is the right time to do this?'. What the participant often means is, 'When is the right time to fight back?' or 'When am I allowed to hit him?', as though they need permission to do their stuff, even when their lives are at stake!

For some reason, women seem to feel that they must justify or explain their actions. The fact that the attacker is in your space is reason enough to launch your defence. You must assess your particular situation. If he's in your house and he's swearing at you or talking to you in a derogatory manner, take action. Don't wait for him to finish his sentence – what he has to say is not important. The fact that he is in your house and in your space is important. He shouldn't be there. When is the best time? When you want to do it – without internal discussion or negotiation happening in your head. You don't need anyone's permission, least of all the attacker's. *Your* permission is permission enough.

Shouting

When you are isolated with your attacker, for instance in a forest where you do not hear voices or music, or see any car lights, do not shout for help. Shouting will achieve nothing and could end up aggravating your attacker, prompting him to knock you out immediately, even kill you.

However, if you are in an area where there are some signs of activity, or you know that there are people close by, shouting could be an effective technique. It is also good to shout while you are executing your techniques – this loud approach will startle your attacker. It will also energize you and help you put more power into your technique. When someone attempts to push a car, they often utter a groan from deep within the throat. A tennis player does the same when attempting a challenging shot. The karate student shouts when executing a technique. It is the combination of power, speed, attitude and determination that achieves the point of focus and ensures success in the application of the technique.

A participant at one of my workshops used to shout 'No!' whenever she applied her techniques. The man that we had enlisted to mock attack her as part of her test was so taken aback every time she shouted that he struggled to focus on the attack and what he was supposed to be doing. This is a wonderful example of how effective shouting can be.

Changing scenarios

It is important to note that each attack situation is different and that, even during the attack, there are continual changes. One woman could be attacked in a dark alley, within close proximity of other people, by a man wielding a knife. Another could be attacked in her home on a small-holding, far away from neighbours, by a man without a weapon. And yet another could be attacked in her work lift where colleagues are working nearby. Each woman has to make a decision about how best to handle her particular situation, bearing in mind that what may be considered an appropriate response in one instance may not be recommended in another.

The continual changes in an attack situation also have to be considered. These changes could be in the form of changing body position, movement, attitude, the changing physical state of the attacker and the woman being attacked, lighting, ground surface, and so on. For example, a rapist may not rape you where he grabs you – he could pull you some distance away to a spot that is less likely to attract attention. He could start off by holding you with both hands, only to release one hand later on. He could be on the left of you and then move to your right. He could release you altogether to open a car door or to undo his zip. So the scene keeps changing. You should not, however, be daunted by these changes. In many cases these changes can be used to your advantage – you simply need to learn to identify them and know how best to use them. I believe that if a person can do different dance steps, such as the cha-cha, rock 'n roll, rumba or two-step, then they can adjust physically in a self-defence scenario by way of rapidly changing body position and methods of counter-attack, for example direct block, shifting between long and short stances, punching, moving out, coming back in to perform yet another punch, and so on.

Your mind and application of self-defence techniques must be flexible enough to adapt to the various changes in the attack, just as the dancer adapts to the various stages of the dance.

The different stages of an attack

The changing scenarios in an attack situation are often referred to as the 'stages of an attack'. An attack can have any number of stages depending on how long and involved the attack is.

Example: You could be standing outside your house, watering the garden. A strange man comes up from behind and grabs your upper body, pinning your arms to your sides (bear-hug position). This is **stage 1** of the attack. He then throws you against the wall or down on the ground. This is **stage 2** of the attack. He grabs your hair and slaps your face. This is **stage 3**. He drops down to the ground and starts strangling you with his one hand. **Stage 4**. With his other hand he starts pulling your pants down. **Stage 5**. And so on. This is what we mean when we say that there are continual changes.

There is a big difference between stage 1 and stage 5. Each stage may or may not offer an opportunity for defence. **The important thing is to recognize the different stages of an attack and to never give up trying to find and take advantage of the gaps presented**. If you weren't able to act at stage 1, there is always stage 2, then stage 3, and so on.

It is obviously recommended that you act as quickly as you can. As mentioned before, you will have the element of surprise on your side. Also bear in mind that, as one stage progresses to the next, there is a real possibility that you will start becoming tired. Being thrown around, hit, pushed, slapped and dragged takes a lot out of you. The less energy you have left and the more injuries you have sustained, the harder it will be to apply your techniques effectively and to maintain the necessary mental and emotional strength required to see you through.

Don't give up! Make your next plan quickly. Adapt. Be flexible. Because each situation is different, it is up to the individual woman concerned to assess her situation and to decide on an appropriate course of action, whether it be to run away, yell, talk her way out of it, or apply self-defence techniques. All of these options are considered 'self-defence'.

The fight (a summary)

If you have been unable to avoid an oncoming attack for whatever reason and are now in a situation where you have to fight back, there are a number of things you should consider.

The rapist's attack can happen in any number of ways: choking, hugging, seizing, holding your arms, grabbing onto your garments, pulling, punching, kicking, pushing or tackling. Do not oppose power with power. Rather apply self-defence techniques to sensitive target areas on his body. For instance, if he has his hands around your throat, don't use your strength to try and pry them off. Apply self-defence techniques with your available arms, hands or legs onto one of his vulnerable body target areas such as the groin, neck, ears or face.

When you apply a self-defence technique, apply it with total focus. There must be no hesitation in your technique or movement. Neither should there be hesitation between your block and counter-attack. Keep your tension alive. Stay concentrated. Don't be nice. Consider all the possibilities necessary to save your life, even if it means spitting into your attacker's face or poking your fingers into his eyes.

Each technique must be performed with the maximum power and speed that you can muster. You must also be sure to focus on the target areas of your attacker's body. If you miss the target area the first time, hit again and again until you DO strike it. If the technique does not work for you, try another, and another, until you are successful. You cannot afford to give up

– you could be fighting for your life. Keep trying until you achieve success. Adapt to the various stages of the fight.

As I've mentioned before, do not drop to the floor voluntarily unless you are confident in self-defence ground techniques. If you are knocked down, get up quickly. Keep your eyes on your attacker at all times and never turn your back on him.

Do not underestimate your attacker and do not trust him, even if he pleads with you. For your own safety, it is better to assume that he could be very powerful with the ability to hurt you, than to naïvely think that he might change his mind and 'take it easy' on you. He has attacked you and this fact alone suggests that he does not care about how you think or feel. Do not give him power by giving him the benefit of the doubt – you are in danger, possibly life-threatening. If you are going to fight back, do so with commitment and strong attitude until your attacker is disabled, dead, unconscious, or you have the opportunity to get away. Remember, your attacker will not forgive your weaknesses.

Take charge of your situation. Take the authority away from your attacker. You are much stronger than you think you are.

Turning crisis into opportunity and identifying advantages

CRISIS	OPPORTUNITY
He's attacking me!	The element of surprise is on my side. He does not expect me to fight back or to use effective self-defence techniques.
He is bigger than me.	I might not be as large as he is, but I can be quicker and more agile. Big tends to be slow. I will use this potential lack of speed to my advantage.
I wake up to find a man standing in my room. It is dark and difficult to see.	I know my room well, even in the dark. He does not. I can move around more easily than he can. I know what objects I can use as potential weapons.

CRISIS	OPPORTUNITY
He is wearing loose, comfortable clothing, but I feel restricted by mine.	I can kick off my high-heel shoes and tear the side of my skirt for movement. Tight clothes are often more difficult to remove. His loose clothing gives me more to grab hold of when applying certain techniques, for example smashing his face onto my knee or performing a knee-technique to his groin. Holding onto him will help me keep my balance.
I wake up to find a naked man at my bedside.	He is an open, vulnerable target. There is no clothing to protect him.
He is making contact with me by grabbing me, strangling me, holding me, etc.	If he is close enough to make contact with me, I am close enough to make contact with him. I can use the opportunity to execute my techniques.
I have been thrown onto a surface of gravel/sand/stones.	I can grab a handful of gravel, sand or stones and throw it hard into his face.
He's hurting me and I feel afraid.	I can hurt him too and I am allowed to hurt him.
I have no weapons.	I still have the element of surprise. There are many things around me that I can use as a weapon – a rolled-up newspaper (jab into throat, face, groin, etc.), a bottle or heavy ceramic flower pot (to hit him over the head), a broom (to hit or jab into his body). I can throw things at him. I have my own body parts as suitable weapons: hands, feet, elbows, knees, legs, etc.
He is intoxicated as well as strong and aggressive.	If he is intoxicated his sense of balance, timing and judgement may be impaired. I can use this to my advantage.

CRISIS	OPPORTUNITY
He looks very threatening.	While you should never underestimate your attacker, this could be his first attempt/attack. If you deal successfully with a first-time attacker, in other words, give him a real hiding, chances are high that he's going to hesitate about attacking again. First-time attackers often experience nervousness and could try to compensate for this by appearing unusually aggressive.
He has a weapon!	While the use of a weapon should never be misjudged or taken lightly, do not empower the attacker so readily just because he has one. He might only use it as a form of intimidation and may not be skilled in its use. (For defence against a weapon, it is advisable to attend a self-defence course to understand the basic platform from which to work. To learn to deal with knife attacks, consider attending a blade-fighting course.)
He is using offensive language and is calling me terrible names. He tells me it's my fault, that I'm to blame!	Don't take what he says personally – it's not important what he thinks. It's NOT your fault and he has absolutely NO right to rape you. Don't allow yourself to be thrown. Stay emotionally strong and committed to what you have to do.
He is physically very strong.	He may be physically strong, but he has sensitive target areas on his body. Hard blows to these areas will hurt him badly, if not immobilize him.
He's very aggressive.	His pattern of attack will determine your response. See pages 30–46 for information on different rape patterns. Keep your wits about you and don't panic.
He smells terrible!	Don't let his odour distract you – stay focused on what you need to do.
He's wearing a suit.	Don't be fooled by appearances!

CRISIS	OPPORTUNITY
He's wearing glasses.	Use his vulnerability to your advantage. He'll certainly use yours against you. Punch his glasses into his eyes or grab them off his face and toss them away; follow up quickly with an effective technique to immobilize him long enough for you to get away.
He has a moustache/beard.	A moustache or beard is a very sensitive target area. Grab hold of it and pull it as hard as you can.
He's wearing a balaclava.	His facial target areas, such as eyes and mouth, are highlighted even more. He's pointing out to you where you should hit!
He's wearing a thick coat.	This gives you more clothing to hang onto when applying certain techniques.
He has a violent, threatening and intimidating approach.	He could be using this approach to create a false sense of ability and proficiency. (Is this just a smokescreen or is his bite really as bad as his bark?) Remember, however, to stay alert at all times.
He's charming, speaks softly, sometimes whispers.	Again, don't be fooled by appearances. Because he appears nice does not mean he *is* nice or can be trusted. There is nothing nice about rape.
He is athletic and physically confident – possibly a sportsperson.	He might not be as coordinated as you would assume. He might not even have good balance (make him move around so that this vulnerability is exposed).

4
BODY TARGET AREAS

Regardless of a man's physical size or build, there are certain areas on his body that are very vulnerable and sensitive. A hard blow or the application of specific techniques to any of these areas can cause fair to extreme pain, immobilization, even death.

In self-defence, the vulnerable and sensitive areas on the body are called the **body target areas**. It is very important to remember these areas because all your self-defence techniques MUST be aimed at your attacker's body target areas for maximum effectiveness. Aiming at the body target areas can make all the difference between a successful technique and an unsuccessful one.

The **most important** body target areas to remember (even if they're the only ones you remember!) are:

- the nose
- the groin
- the throat
- the back of the neck

Thereafter:

- the eyes
- the ears
- the upper back
- the fingers
- the point of the chin
- the solar plexus.

BODY TARGET AREAS

BODY FROM THE BACK

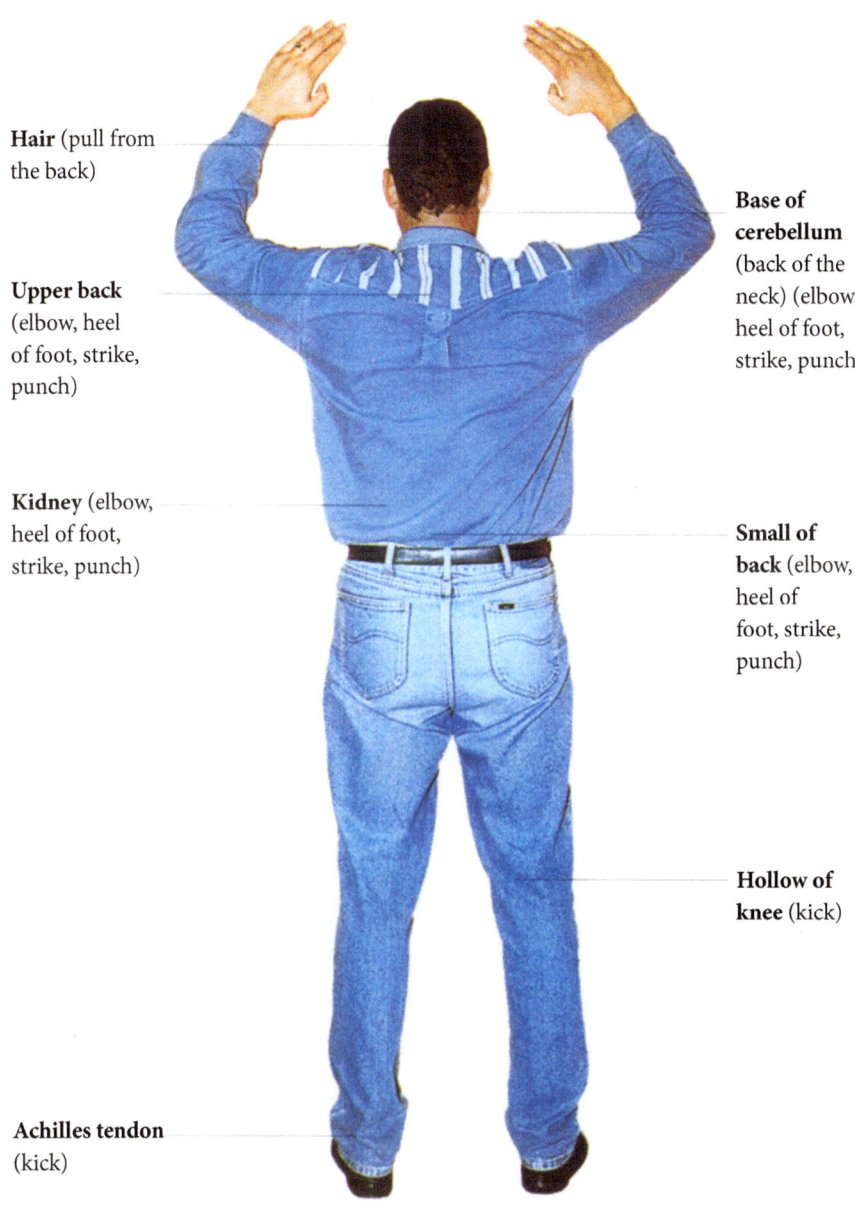

Hair (pull from the back)

Upper back (elbow, heel of foot, strike, punch)

Kidney (elbow, heel of foot, strike, punch)

Base of cerebellum (back of the neck) (elbow, heel of foot, strike, punch)

Small of back (elbow, heel of foot, strike, punch)

Hollow of knee (kick)

Achilles tendon (kick)

BODY FROM THE FRONT

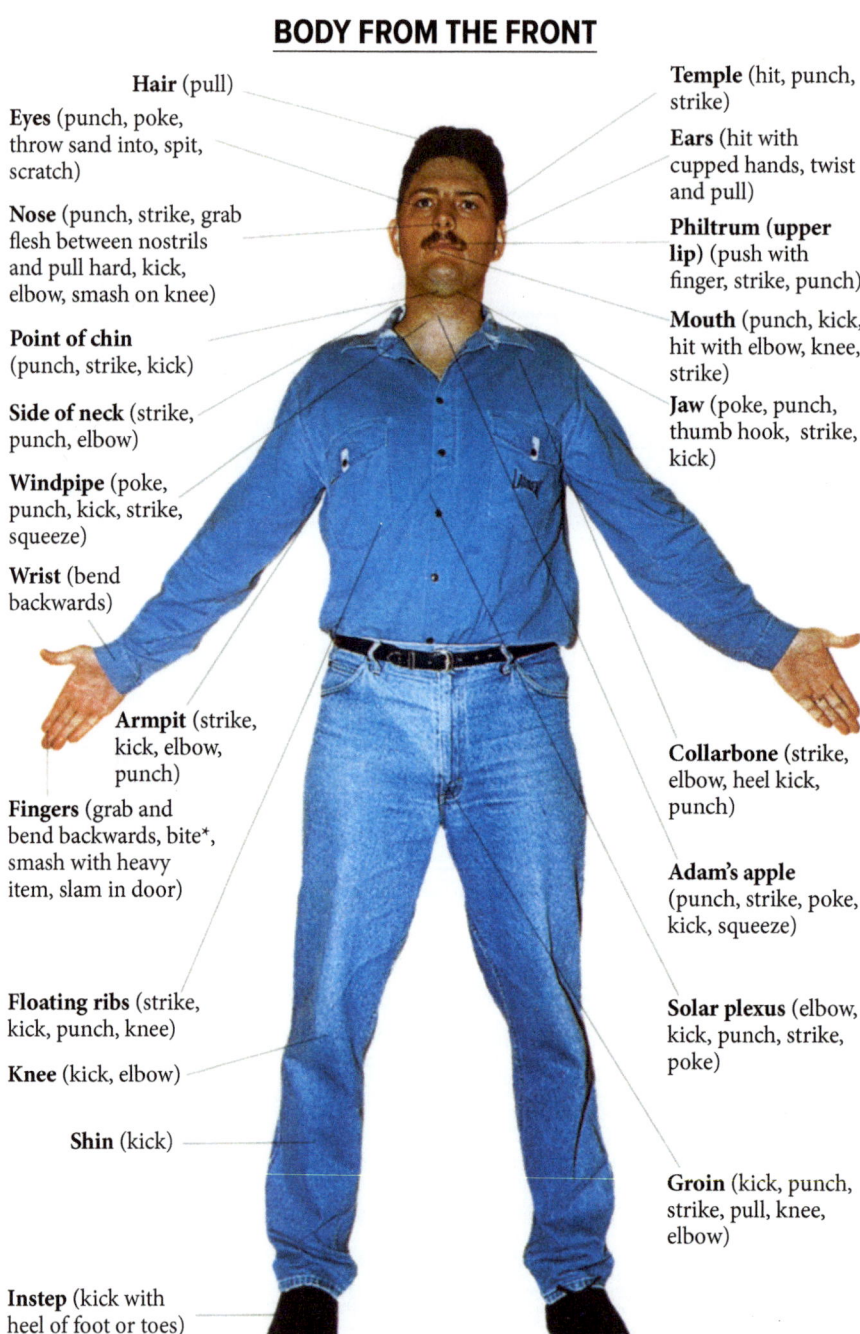

Hair (pull)

Eyes (punch, poke, throw sand into, spit, scratch)

Nose (punch, strike, grab flesh between nostrils and pull hard, kick, elbow, smash on knee)

Point of chin (punch, strike, kick)

Side of neck (strike, punch, elbow)

Windpipe (poke, punch, kick, strike, squeeze)

Wrist (bend backwards)

Armpit (strike, kick, elbow, punch)

Fingers (grab and bend backwards, bite*, smash with heavy item, slam in door)

Floating ribs (strike, kick, punch, knee)

Knee (kick, elbow)

Shin (kick)

Instep (kick with heel of foot or toes)

Temple (hit, punch, strike)

Ears (hit with cupped hands, twist and pull)

Philtrum (upper lip) (push with finger, strike, punch)

Mouth (punch, kick, hit with elbow, knee, strike)

Jaw (poke, punch, thumb hook, strike, kick)

Collarbone (strike, elbow, heel kick, punch)

Adam's apple (punch, strike, poke, kick, squeeze)

Solar plexus (elbow, kick, punch, strike, poke)

Groin (kick, punch, strike, pull, knee, elbow)

Foot (stamp)

5
BASIC SELF-DEFENCE TECHNIQUES

INTRODUCTION

Self-defence techniques are the individual elements that make up a self-defence pattern or sequence. Each pattern or sequence can consist of a number of techniques, executed individually or in combination.

To become proficient at applying self-defence techniques, I recommend that you slowly run through each of the self-defence techniques until you feel reasonably familiar with the movement and process. I also suggest that you work with a partner. This will help you to accurately judge distance and will provide you with real target areas. Try to make slight contact (touch) with these areas when practicing your techniques. Before you start, it is best to do a short warm-up and stretch to prevent injury.

Start building up speed and power, still aiming for the sensitive target areas. Your techniques should be a lot faster and stronger. Keep practicing and building on your techniques in this way until you feel more confident and your responses become automatic. It is well worth making the effort with these techniques because they are something that you can take with you wherever you go. They are always easily accessible and they're YOURS!

Adopting a stance (fighting stance)

Adopting a good, balanced stance is important for three reasons. Firstly, it enables you to be **ready** and in a suitable position to execute your techniques. It also means you'll be ready for any techniques your attacker directs at you. Secondly, it provides **good balance** so that you can execute your techniques more effectively, and it enables you to better handle the strikes and blows thrown by your attacker. Thirdly, it enables you to quickly **shift** out of the way of incoming blows from your attacker and allow you, in turn, to more easily shift your body to execute your own techniques.

A fighting stance is an effective stance to use as a platform for launching techniques and for returning to whenever you are not in motion, or when you have completed a sequence of techniques.

1 Stand with one foot in front of the other, approximately shoulder-width apart.

2 Your feet should be pointing in the direction you are facing (the direction of the attacker).

3 Bend your front knee and lock your back leg.

4 Lift your arms into a fighting position, clenching both fists. Keep your head up and look the attacker in the eye.

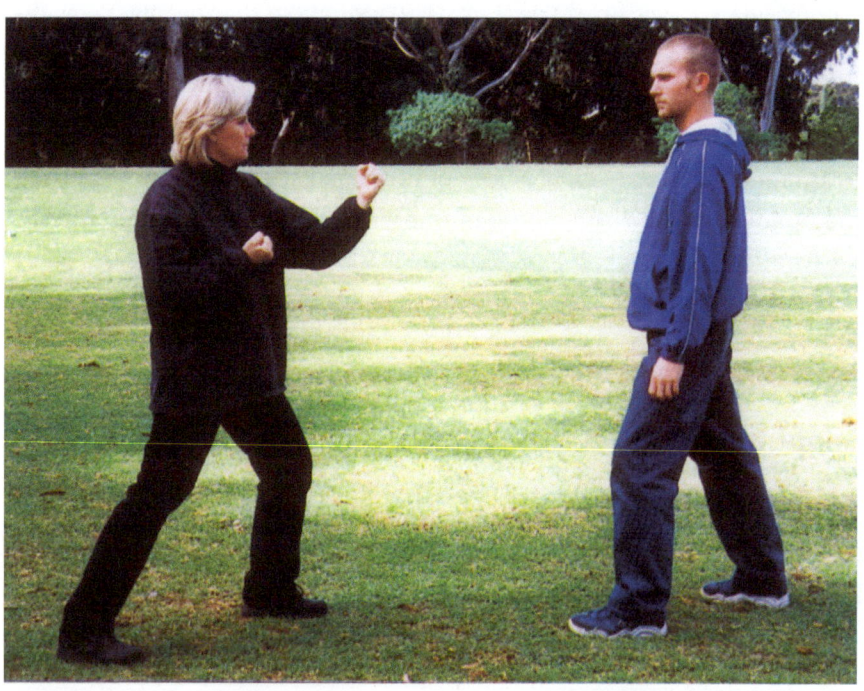

BASIC SELF-DEFENCE TECHNIQUES

Maintaining proper distance

There are three basic ranges of distance in self-defence: **1** Close range, **2** medium range, and **3** long range.

All self-defence techniques have a range within which they are most effective. While some techniques will simply be ineffective if not implemented within the correct range, other techniques cannot be implemented at all if the range is incorrect. Moving between different ranges involves shifting your body. You can either move your body towards your attacker or away from him to establish the correct distance for your techniques.

Looking at the techniques illustrated below, you will easily see which are short, medium and long-range techniques.

1 Short range.
This is where close-up techniques are executed, for example punches, elbow techniques, knee-jabs, strikes, etc.

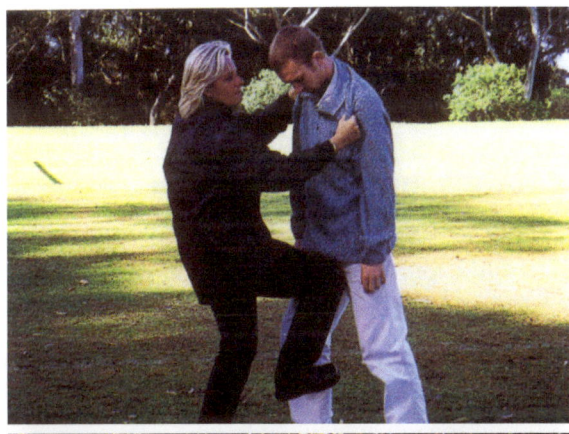

2 Medium range.
This is the correct distance for kicking.

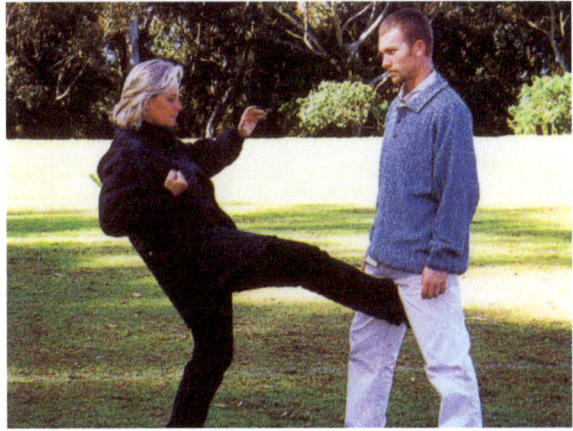

3 Long range.
This range provides a safe distance between you and your assailant. In order to execute a technique, you would have to shift or slide quickly into medium or short range. NEVER kick when standing at long range – your foot can easily be caught.

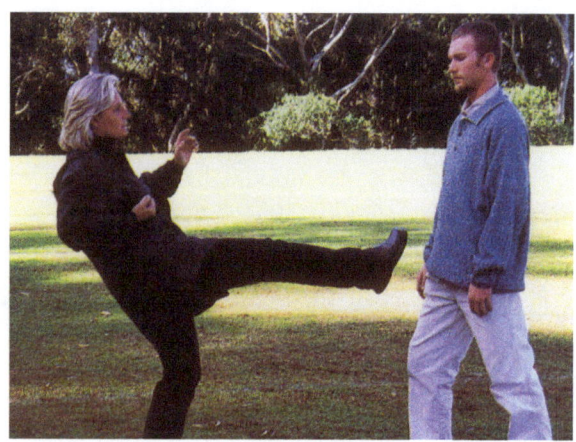

Shifting as a defence

Shifting can be used instead of blocking or in conjunction with blocking (see Basic blocking, pages 79–80). In other words, you can shift *or* you can shift and block at the same time. There are seven basic ways of shifting: forwards, backwards, to the left of the attacker, to the right of the attacker, right around the attacker until you are standing behind him, pivoting (on the balls of your feet), and dropping to the ground to do a ground technique (not advisable for beginners).

Shifting your body is very important, especially if you see the attacker moving in to attack you. Quickly shifting backwards will help break his body force and the impact will be softer.

Remember, your feet are not nailed to the ground. Move them. Failing to do so is the equivalent of standing in front of an oncoming bus and letting it drive over you!

BASIC SELF-DEFENCE TECHNIQUES

1 You can move your body sideways, to the left, out of the line of attack.

2 You can move your body sideways, to the right, out of the line of attack.

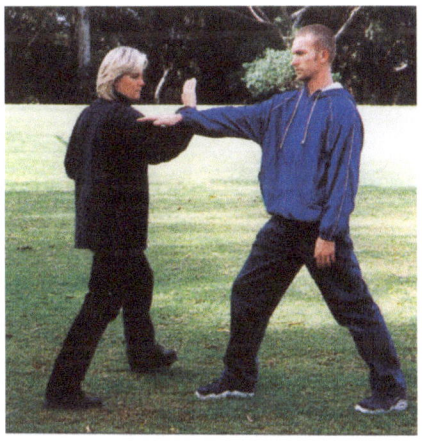

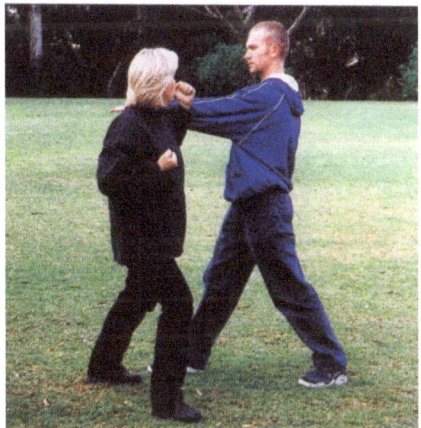

3 When your attacker moves forward, you can move your body backwards to maintain a safe distance.

4 When your attacker moves backwards, you can move your body forwards to re-establish a safe, yet 'workable' distance from which to launch your technique.

5 You can get around and behind your attacker by:
» shifting to the left;
» moving forward;
» passing the side of your attacker;
» turning your body around to face him and
» shifting your feet and body so that you are directly behind him.

How to make a fist

1 Open your hand and place your fingers together.

2 Roll your fingers up into your hand.

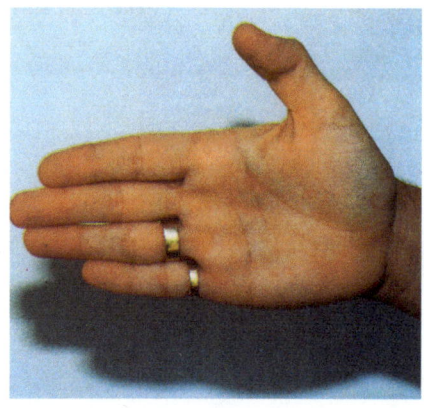

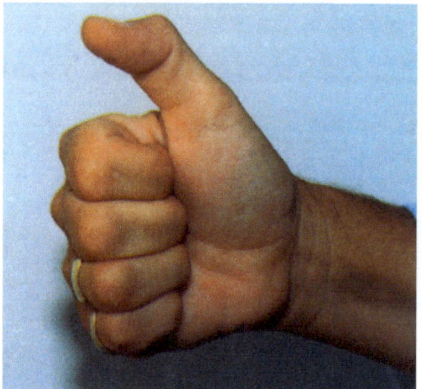

3 Place your thumb over your clenched fingers. Tighten your fist.

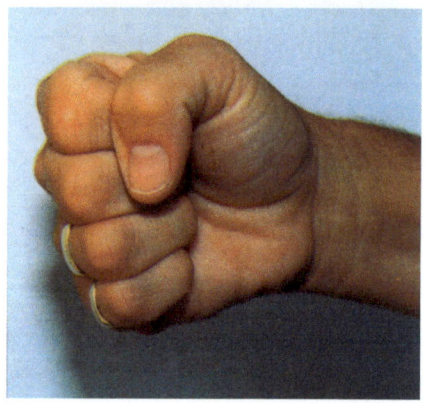

Punching

It's a good idea to invest in a punching pad (available from most major sports stores). A punching pad enables you to practice your punching whilst gauging your power and speed at the same time. This will give you a more accurate idea of how powerful your punches are and how effective they'll be against your assailant. A punching pad also enables you to get used to the feel of the technique and to build confidence in your punching. It will teach you that making hard impact is okay.

BASIC SELF-DEFENCE TECHNIQUES

1 Make a fist.

2 Punch towards the pad.

3 If you just touch the pad with your arm fully extended, you are standing too far from the pad. When you connect with the pad, your arm should still be slightly bent. This means that when faced with a real attacker and applying your punch with full force, it will have more impact.

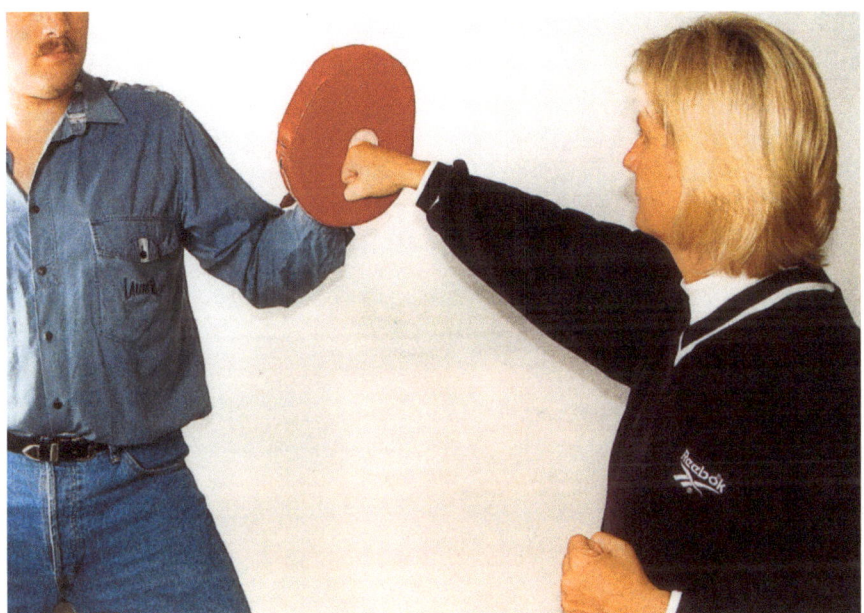

Kicking

Kicking pads are also available and are invaluable in helping you gauge proper distance, power and accuracy. With a bit of practice you will be able to improve your balance and technique, both during and after the kick. There are a few basic things to remember:

» Pull your foot back so that you kick with the **ball** of your foot (when kicking against a pad while wearing shoes, the toe of the shoe may be used).
» Lift your knee. If you are kicking into the groin, point your knee in the direction of the groin. Your foot will land in the direction that your knee is pointing. The higher you lift your knee, the higher the kick will be. The lower your knee, the lower the kick.
» Kick out your foot, connect with the target, and **quickly snap it back** towards your body (snap kick), to prevent the attacker grabbing your foot.

The important thing to remember when practicing kicks is to do them as accurately and as powerfully as possible.

1 Stand in a fighting stance.

2 Bring your leg up for a kick and try to land the kick on the pad.
Note: Your foot will land in the direction your knee is pointing. The higher you lift your knee, the higher you can land your kick. Bring your foot back as quickly as possible to prevent your attacker grabbing hold of it.

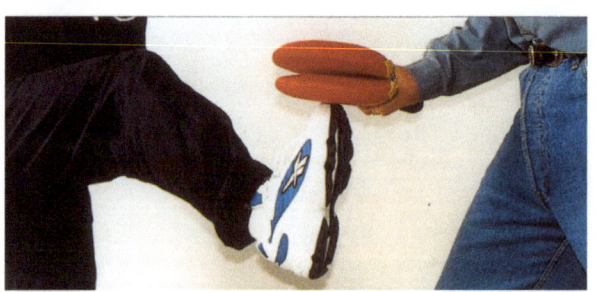

3 Immediately resume your fighting stance.

BASIC SELF-DEFENCE TECHNIQUES

Wind up

Most blocks, punches, strikes, elbow techniques, knee techniques and so on, will be preceded by a quick wind up. A wind up is simply a movement that creates a longer distance for the technique to travel so that it can gather maximum speed (momentum) and force. A good wind up helps generate a fast and strong technique.

A wind up normally involves moving your arm or leg in the opposite direction to which it will eventually be directed. In other words, to do an elbow strike downwards, your wind up will involve first lifting your arm and elbow upwards, before changing direction to move downwards hard.

Basic blocking

Blocking is a technique used to block or deflect oncoming blows. You will need to block if you haven't been able to shift out of the way of an oncoming technique. You may even need to use a block as well as shift your body out of the way. There are a variety of blocks, but the two most frequently used have been featured here.

1 Upper block (defending your face).
Bend your arm to form a 135° angle at the inner elbow. Raise your elbow upwards to slightly above your forehead in a 'pushing' action. Your arm should maintain the 135° angle at the inner elbow.

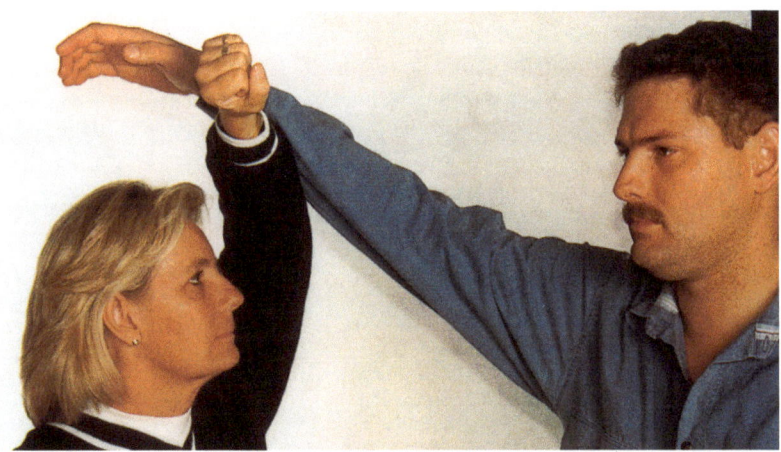

THE SOUTH AFRICAN WOMEN'S GUIDE TO SELF-DEFENCE

2. **Downward block (defending your chest, stomach and groin area).**
Bend your arm and place your hand at your ear, keeping your elbow close to your body (this is the wind up). Then, swing your arm downward and slightly away from your body.

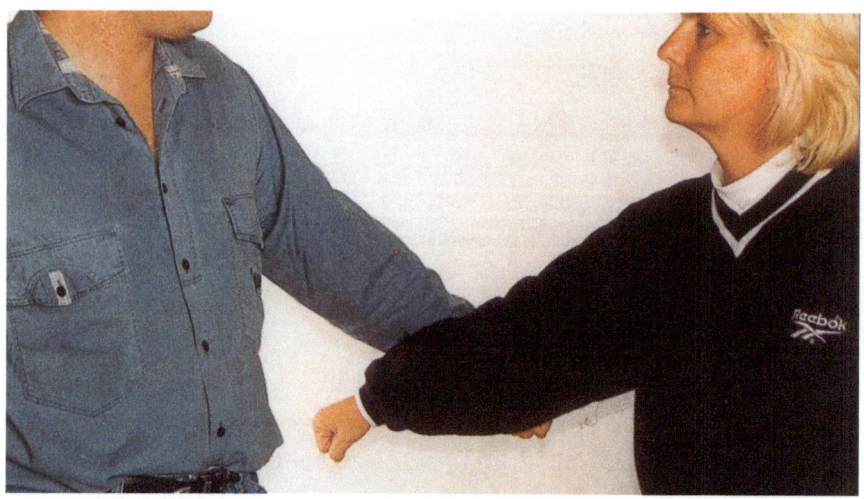

APPLYING BASIC TECHNIQUES ONTO THE TARGET AREAS

HAND AND ARM TECHNIQUES TO THE FACE AND NECK

1. **Finger push.**
Place finger between the upper lip and nostril. Push backwards hard.

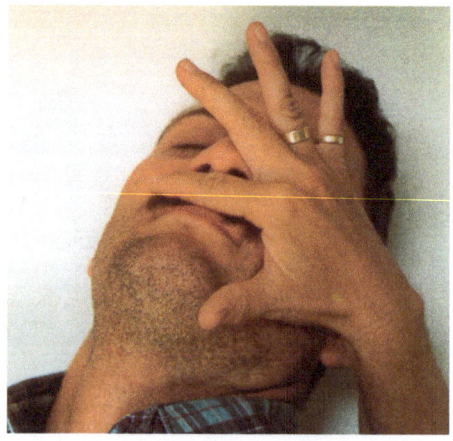

BASIC SELF-DEFENCE TECHNIQUES

2 Thumb-hook under jaw. Hook thumb in and under the jaw. Push backwards hard.

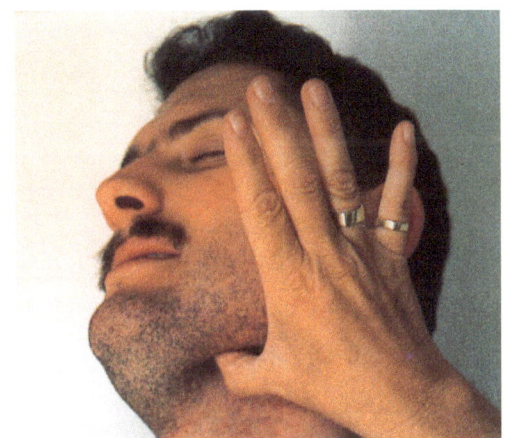

3 Palm-heel strike to nose. Open your hand and place your fingers together as though to make a fist. Pull your fingers backwards and strike (hit) the nose, preferably from just underneath it with the palm-heel of your hand.

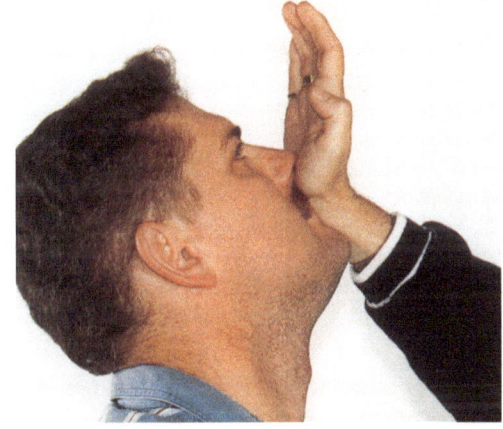

4 Palm-heel strike under jaw. Make a palm-heel striking hand as before and strike hard under the jaw.

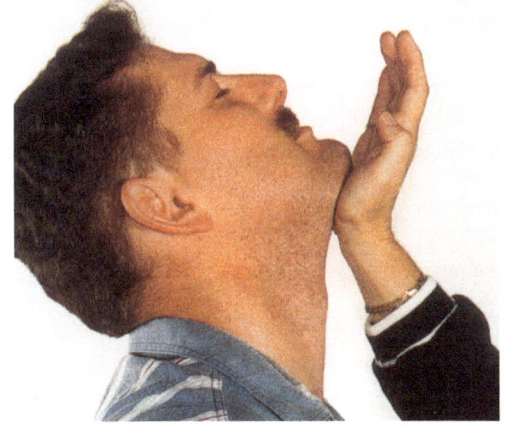

THE SOUTH AFRICAN WOMEN'S GUIDE TO SELF-DEFENCE

5. **Hair pull.** Grab hair as close to the scalp as possible and pull hard.

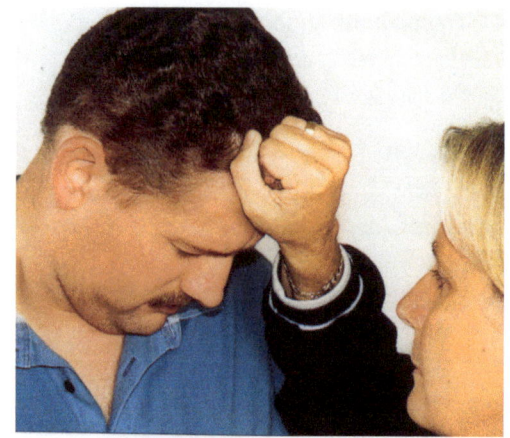

6. **Cupped-hand technique.** Open your hands and place your fingers together. Then, with fingers still together, cup your hands to form 'cymbals'. Hit the ears (in the same motion as playing cymbals). This technique can burst the attacker's ear drums.

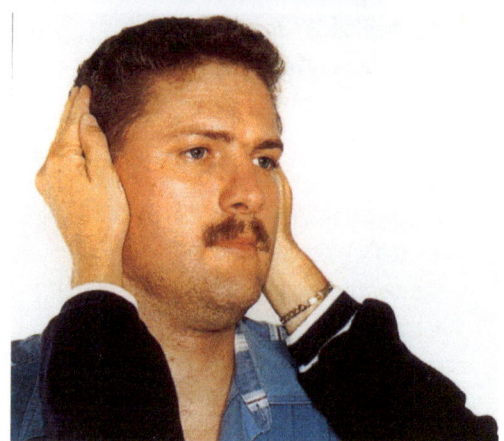

7. **Hammerfist.** Make a fist. Hit hard with the inner part of your clenched fist in an anti-clockwise direction onto the temple. (If you are left-handed, hit in a clockwise direction.)

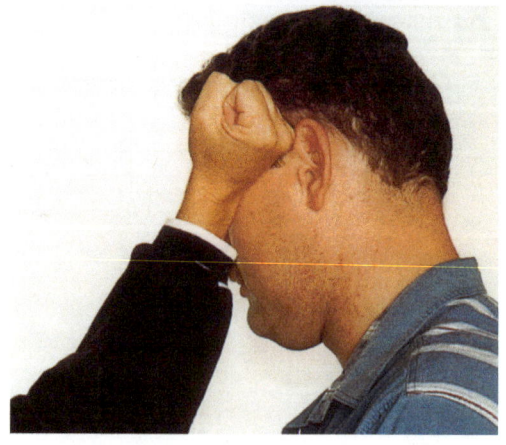

BASIC SELF-DEFENCE TECHNIQUES

8 Finger poke. Poke both of your thumbs into your attacker's eyes. You can also use the index and middle fingers of one hand by straightening them out and spreading them apart into a V-shape.

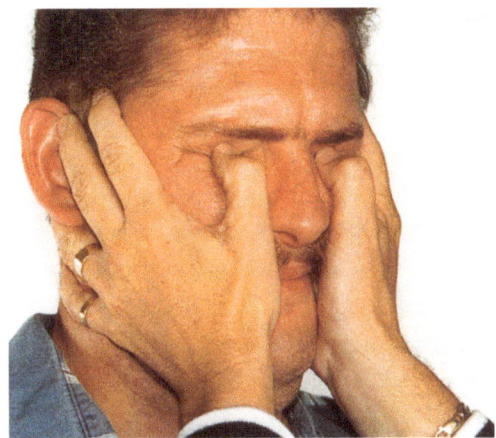

9 Punch to nose. Make a fist as described on page 76 and punch the nose hard.

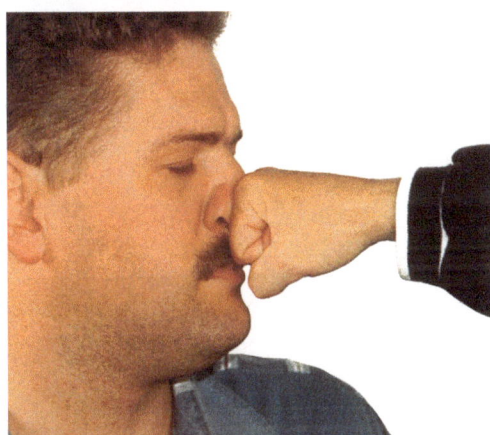

10 Punch to mouth. Make a fist and punch the mouth hard.

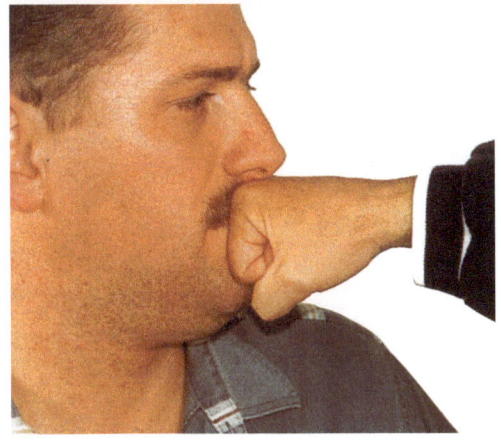

11 **Punch to chin.** Make a fist and punch the chin hard.

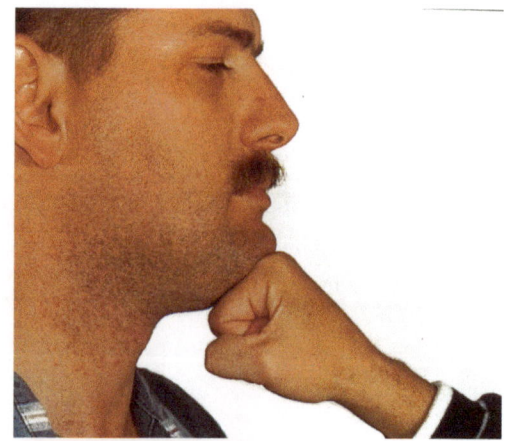

12 **Punch to throat.** Make a fist and punch the throat hard.

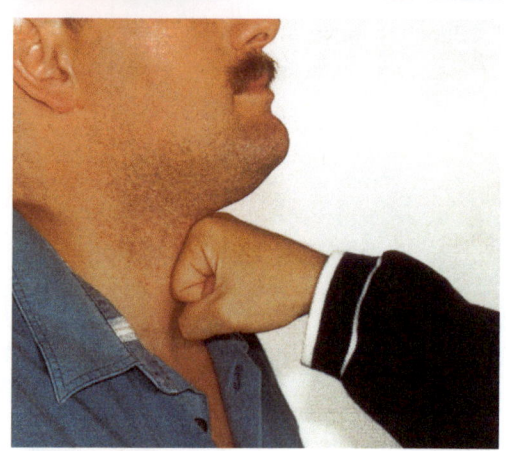

13 **Elbow strike under jaw.** Make an elbow by bending your arm completely. Then, starting with your elbow pointing towards the ground, lift it up high and fast to connect under your attacker's chin (like an upper-cut).

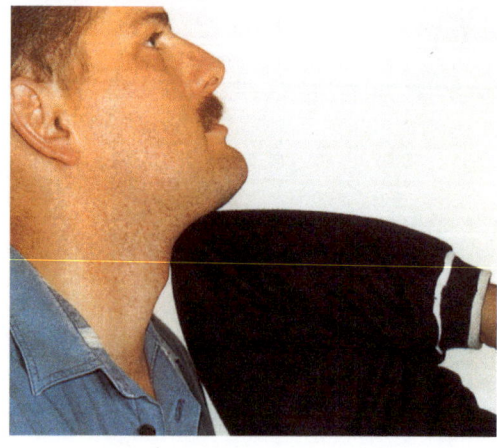

BASIC SELF-DEFENCE TECHNIQUES

14 Elbow strike to the jaw. Make an elbow as before, but wind up by swinging your elbow back behind your body, then bring it forwards hard and fast towards the side of your attacker's chin.

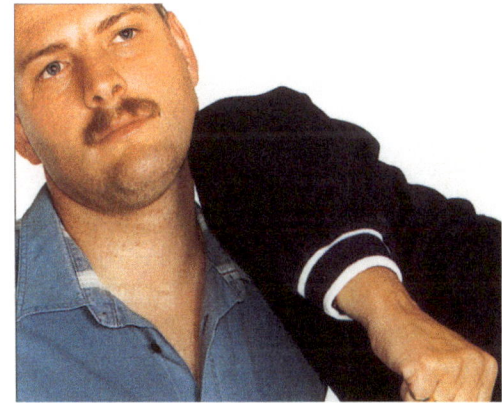

15 Chop to upper lip. Open your hand and place your fingers together. With your palm facing downwards, strike (chop) with the side of your hand (not the fingers) between the upper lip and nostrils.

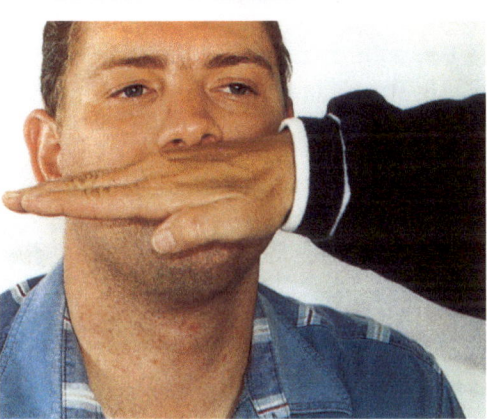

16 Ear grab and twist. Grab the ear tightly. Twist and pull.

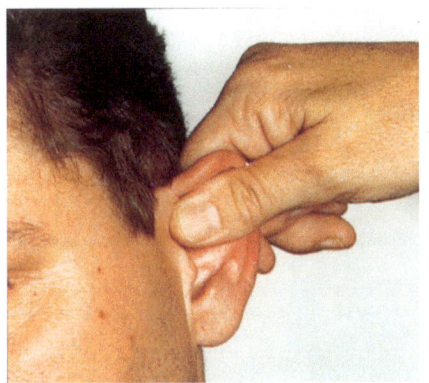
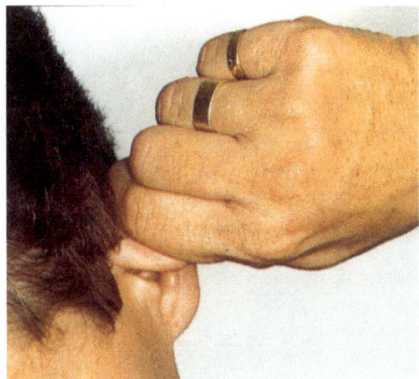

THE SOUTH AFRICAN WOMEN'S GUIDE TO SELF-DEFENCE

17 Spear strike to throat. Open your hand and place your fingers together. Strike the throat target area below the Adam's apple hard with your fingers pointed.

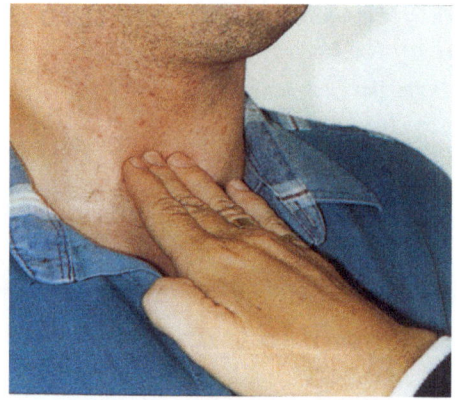

18 Chop to throat. Open your hand and place your fingers together. Strike hard with the side of your hand (not the fingers) onto the throat.

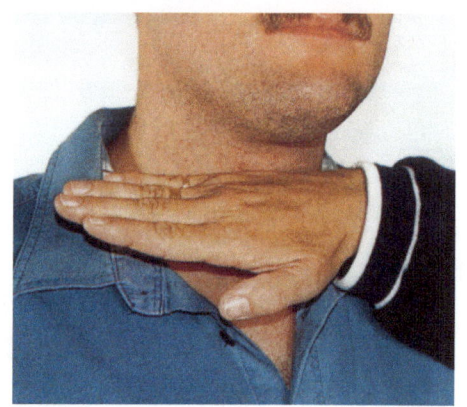

19 Chop to neck. Open your hand and place your fingers together. Strike hard with the side of your hand (not the fingers) onto the side of the neck.

a) Chop to neck with wrist pointing up.   b) Chop to neck with wrist pointing down.

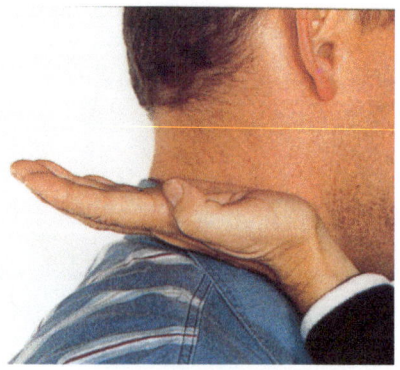 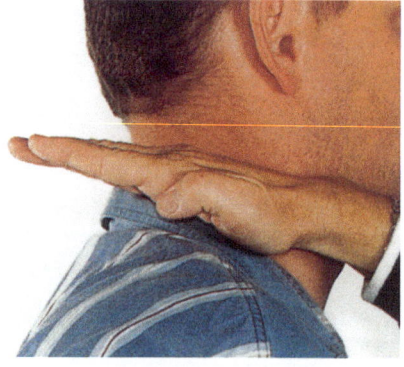

BASIC SELF-DEFENCE TECHNIQUES

HAND AND ARM TECHNIQUES TO THE FRONT OF THE BODY

1 **Elbow strike to collarbone.**
Wind up by lifting your elbow high in the air, then bring it down hard onto the collarbone.

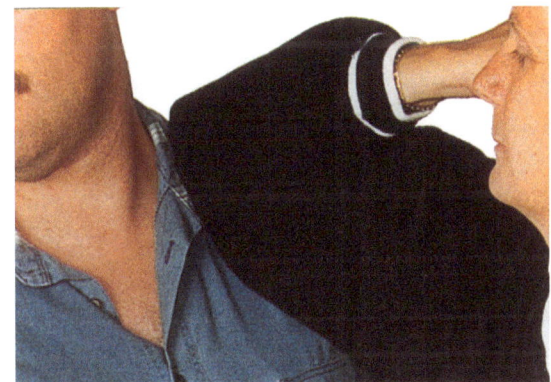

2 **Elbow strike to armpit.**
Wind up by lifting elbow in the air, then bring it down hard and in a forward movement onto the armpit. Or, wind up by taking your elbow back and to the side and, with a sideways motion, swing your arm into the armpit.

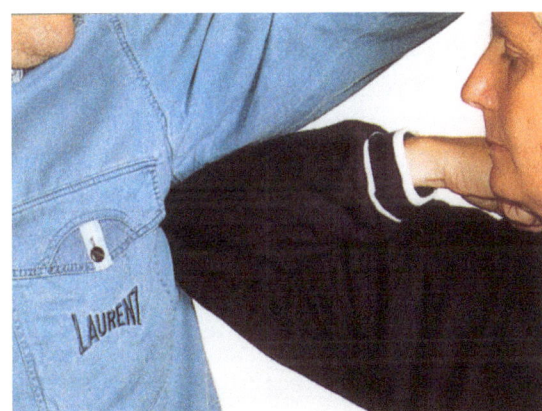

3 **Elbow strike to solar plexus.**
If your attacker is standing, wind up with a sideways motion and swing your arm around into the solar plexus. If your attacker is on his back, your wind up will be from above his body, down onto his solar plexus.

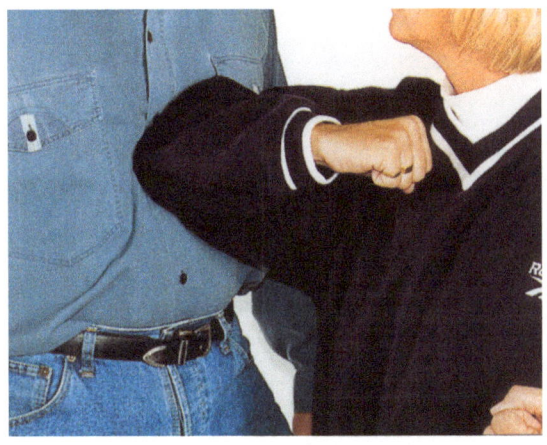

4. **Elbow strike to ribs.** If your attacker is standing, wind up with a sideways motion and swing your arm around and into his ribs. If your attacker is on his back, your wind up will be from above his body, down onto his ribs.

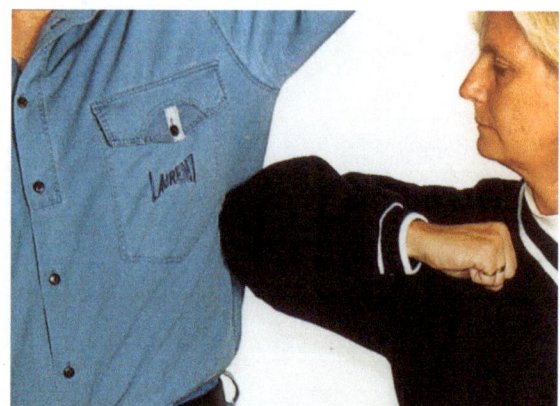

5. **Elbow strike to groin.** Drop your body so that your attacker's groin is in line with your raised elbow. Wind up with a sideways motion across your body and release the elbow strike by swinging your arm backwards and into his groin. To add power to this technique, you can grasp the hand of the arm executing the technique with your other hand and use the power from both arms to drive in the technique.

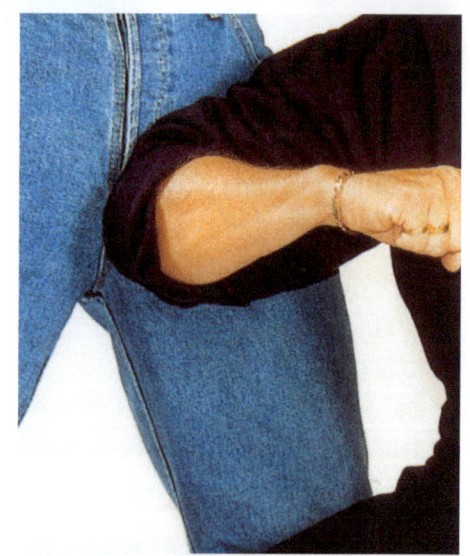

6. **Arm strike to groin.** Make a fist. Wind up with your fist close to your chest. Strike downwards hard with your arm into your attacker's groin.

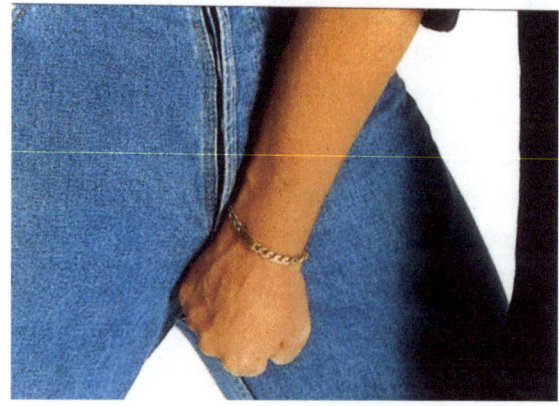

BASIC SELF-DEFENCE TECHNIQUES

7 Fist strike to groin. Make a fist. Wind up with your fist close to your chest. Strike downwards hard with the back of your fist into your attacker's groin.

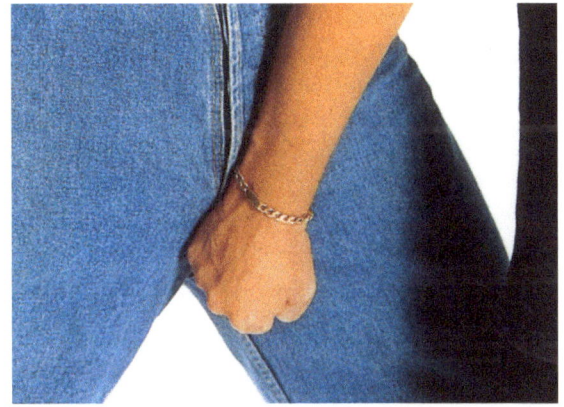

8 Chop to groin. Open your hand and place your fingers together. Strike with the side of your hand (not the fingers) downwards hard onto the groin.

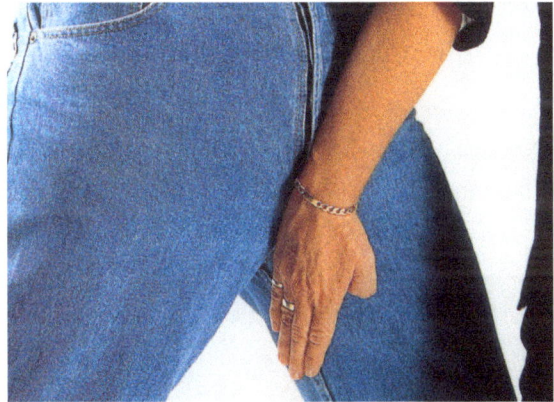

9 Palm-heel strike to groin. Open your hand and place your fingers together as though to make a fist, wrist pointing up. Pull your fingers backwards and strike the groin hard with the heel of your palm.

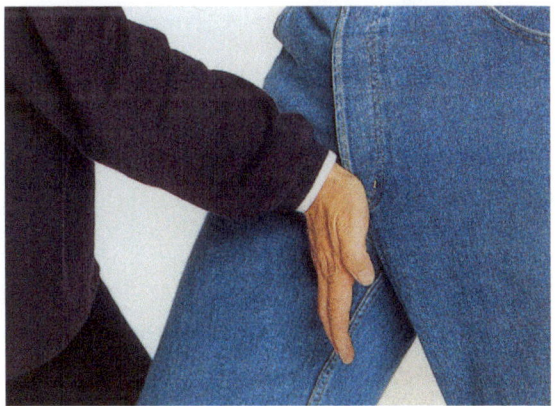

THE SOUTH AFRICAN WOMEN'S GUIDE TO SELF-DEFENCE

10 Grab to the groin. Grab the groin. Squeeze tightly or pull.

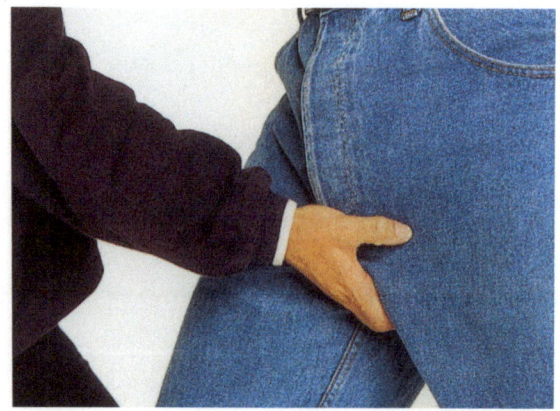

HAND AND ARM TECHNIQUES TO THE BACK OF THE BODY

1 Double-hand strike to back of neck. Clench your hands tightly together. Lift your hands above your head as a wind up and bring them down hard onto the back of the attacker's neck.

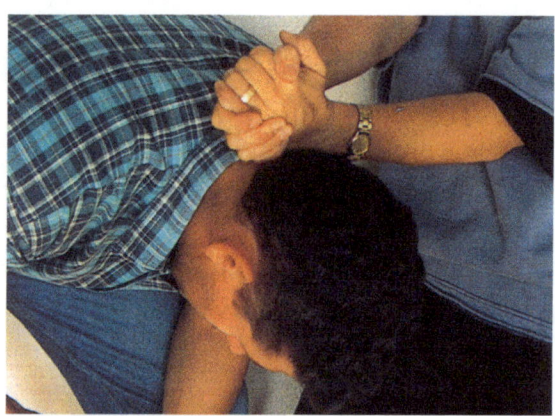

2 Elbow strike to back of neck. Wind up by lifting your elbow high up into the air, then bring it down hard onto the back of the attacker's neck.

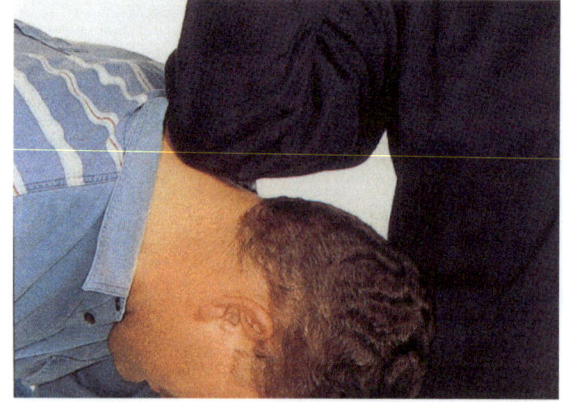

BASIC SELF-DEFENCE TECHNIQUES

3 Elbow strike between shoulder blades.
Wind up by lifting your elbow high into the air, then bring it down hard onto the area between the attacker's shoulder blades.

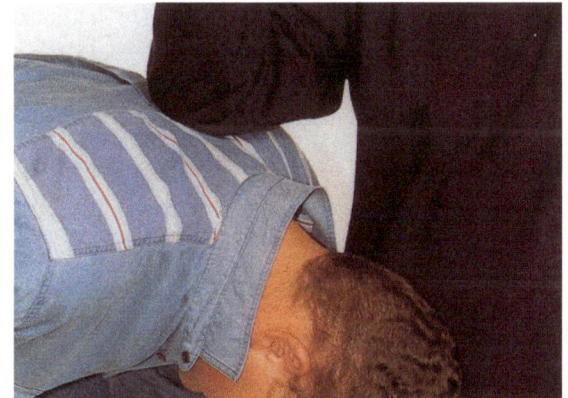

4 Elbow strike to lower back.
Wind up with a sideways motion across your body and release the elbow strike by swinging your arm backwards and into his lower back. To add power to this technique, you can grasp the hand of the arm executing the technique with your other hand and use the power from both arms to drive in the technique.

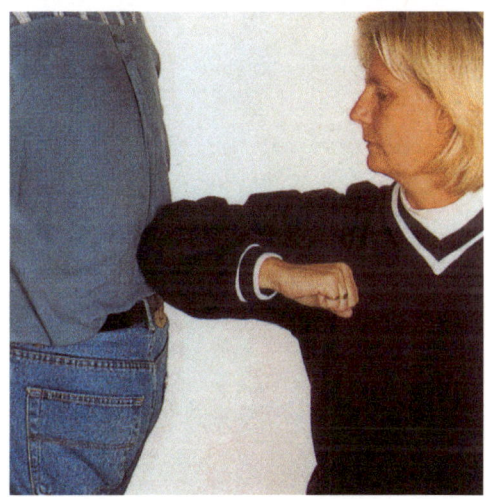

WRIST AND SPECIAL HAND TECHNIQUES

1 Gooseneck-grip.
Stand next to the assailant. Place your arm between his arm and his body. Grip his hand tightly with your hand while holding onto his arm with your other hand. Bend his hand down.

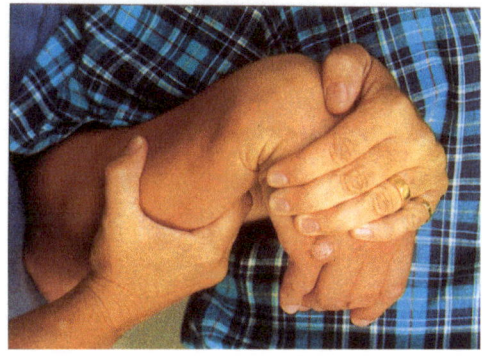

2 Finger twist.
Hold on tightly to your assailant's little finger and bend it backwards.

3 Knuckle strike.
Make a tight fist. Push the knuckle of your middle finger outwards. Turn your hand so that the knuckle is pointing down and strike hard onto the top of your attacker's hand.

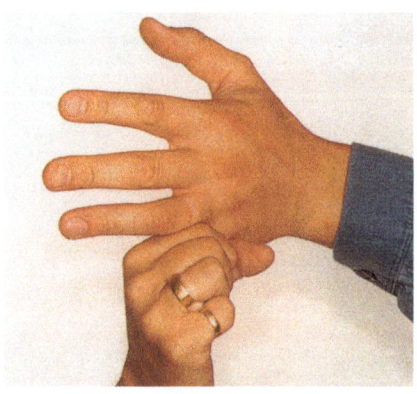
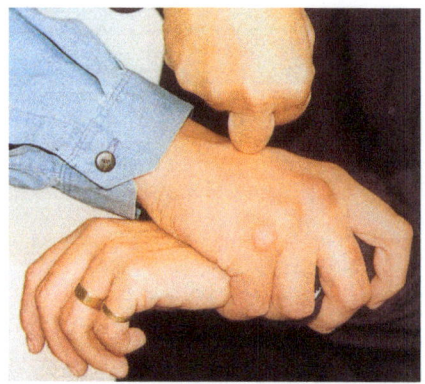

KICKING AND LEG TECHNIQUES

1 Knee-jab to face.
Holding your attacker to aid your balance, bring your knee up hard and onto his nose.

2 Knee-jab to groin.
Holding your attacker to aid your balance, bring your knee up hard and into his groin.

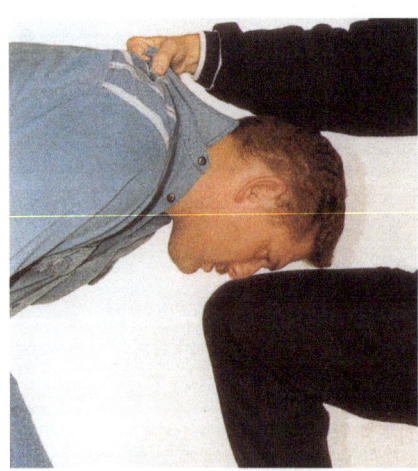
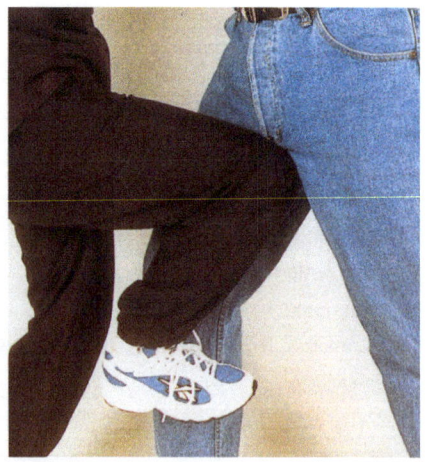

BASIC SELF-DEFENCE TECHNIQUES

3 Kick to groin.
Pull your foot back, bend your knee and snap kick with your foot into his groin.

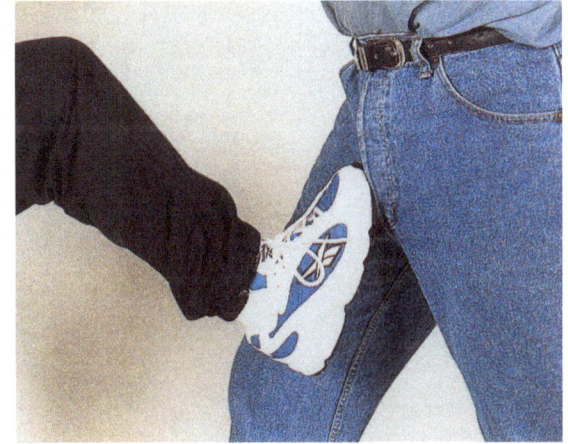

4 Leg swing to groin.
Swing your leg upwards and between your assailant's legs, into his groin.

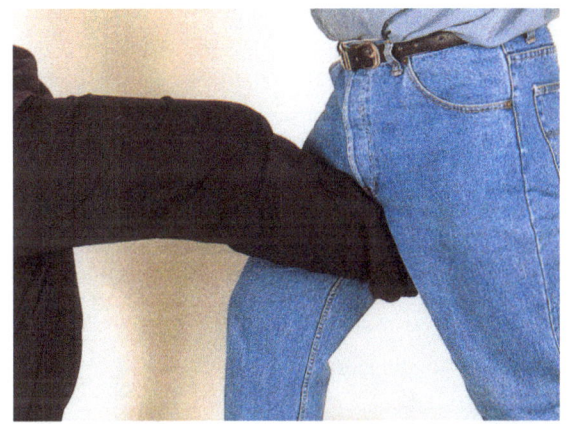

5 Kick to kneecap.
Pull your foot back slightly and give a hard kick to the knee.

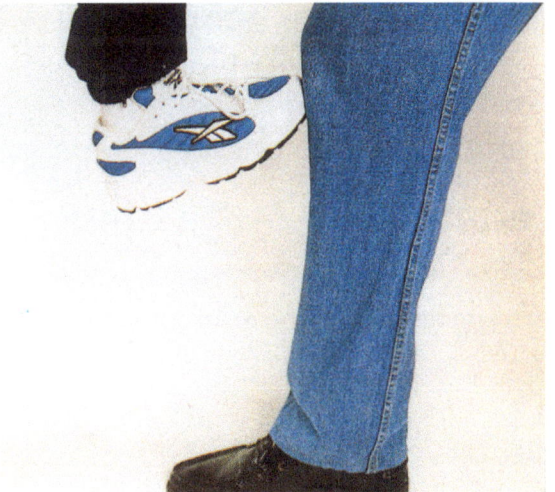

THE SOUTH AFRICAN WOMEN'S GUIDE TO SELF-DEFENCE

6 Kick to shin. Pull your foot back slightly and give a hard kick to the shin.

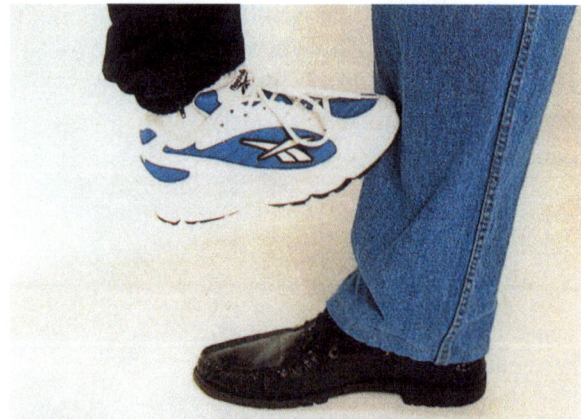

7 Rear kick to groin. Pull your foot back and kick from behind, up between your assailant's legs and into his groin.

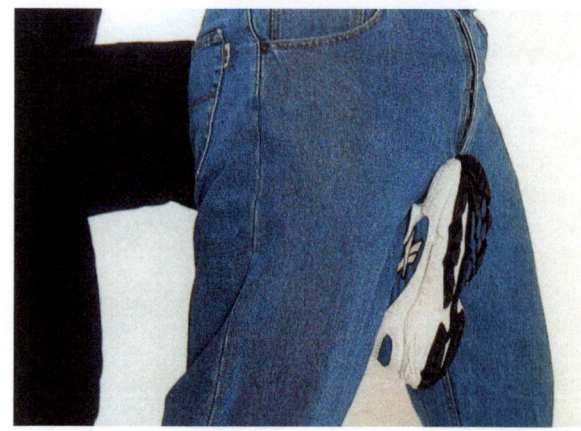

8 Downward kick to back of knee. Lift up your knee and, using the side of your foot, kick down hard onto the back of the knee.

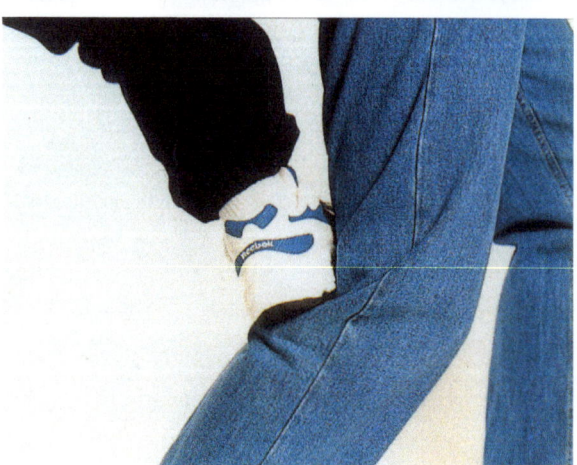

BASIC SELF-DEFENCE TECHNIQUES

9 Downward kick to side of knee.

Lift up your knee and, using the side of your foot, kick down hard onto the side of the knee.

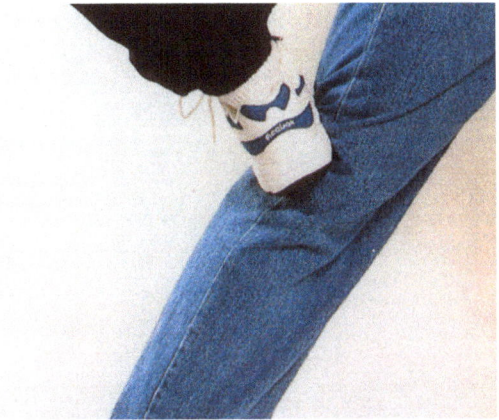

10 Kick on Achilles tendon.

Give a hard kick onto the Achilles tendon

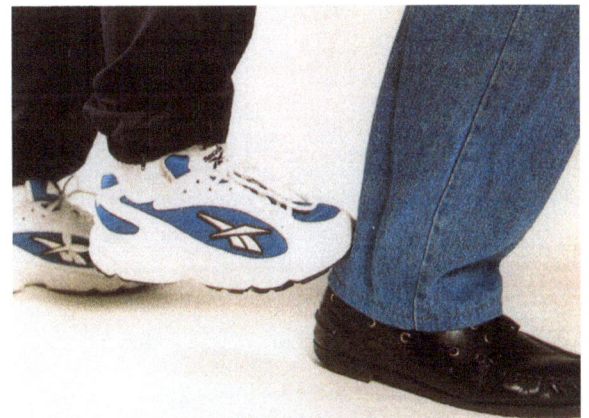

11 Kick to foot.

Using the heel of your foot, stamp down hard onto the bridge of your assailant's foot or onto his toes.

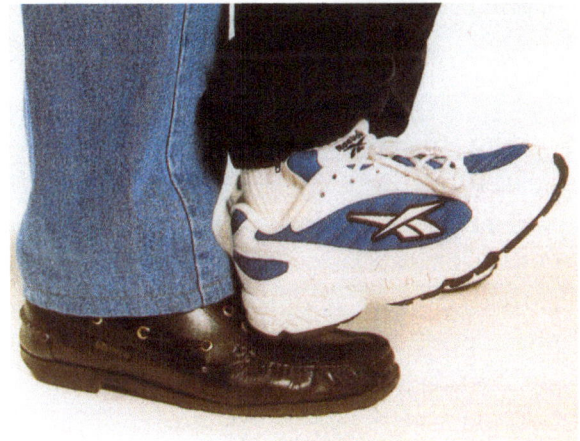

6
SELF-DEFENCE SCENARIOS

All the scenarios presented in this section have been well tested. Reading this book on its own is not going to make you proficient at self-defence, although it will increase your awareness, motivate you, create the mind shift necessary for self-defence and offer options that you may never have thought of before. However, I cannot stress strongly enough how important it is to actually practice your techniques in order to master them, preferably with a partner.

After you have run through and practiced all the basic self-defence techniques illustrated in the previous chapter, you will be ready to begin applying these techniques to simulated attack scenarios.

Due to the technical nature of a few of the techniques presented here, we have highlighted them (using the 🧍🧍 icon) as techniques that must be practiced with a friend or partner first.

As with the self-defence techniques, each of these scenarios should first be done slowly in order to understand the application of the techniques and to be sure that the techniques are being done correctly within the framework of the individual scenario. You should then start practicing them using maximum power and speed, because this is how you'll have to do it if ever faced by an attacker.

An important point to remember is that, in real life, an attack is not an organized, predictable event. If a specific technique is not working for you after trying it at least three times, don't persist. Move on to plan B, then plan C, and so on. The scenarios presented here are guidelines. Should you have to deviate from them because your situation suddenly changes, adapt and do something else.

SELF-DEFENCE SCENARIOS

> **GOLDEN RULE:**
> Apply basic techniques onto available and open body target areas.
> Be flexible and keep an open mind.

ATTACKS FROM THE FRONT

ATTACK TO THE THROAT WITH BOTH HANDS (1)

Because 90% of all attacks occur with a strike or some other action to the upper body area (strangling being frequently noted), this technique is ideal for an attack of this nature. Your assailant's groin is within easy reach and you can use any solid surface behind you, such as a wall or car, to help support you if necessary while executing your first technique.

1 Your assailant approaches as you are getting into your car.

2 If you hear your assailant approach, quickly turn around to face him.

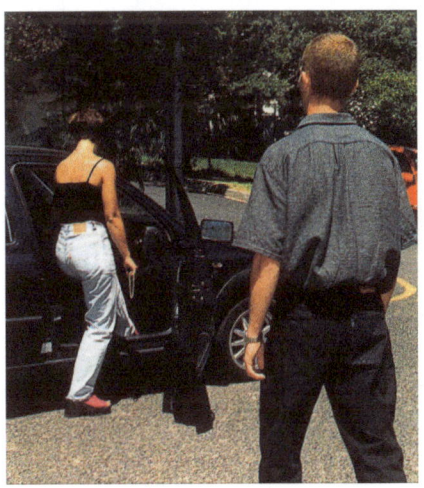
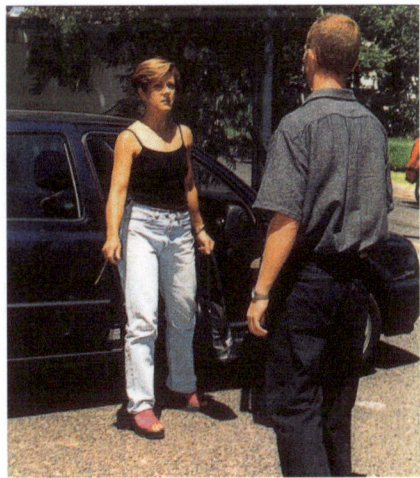

3 Your assailant grabs your throat with both his hands.

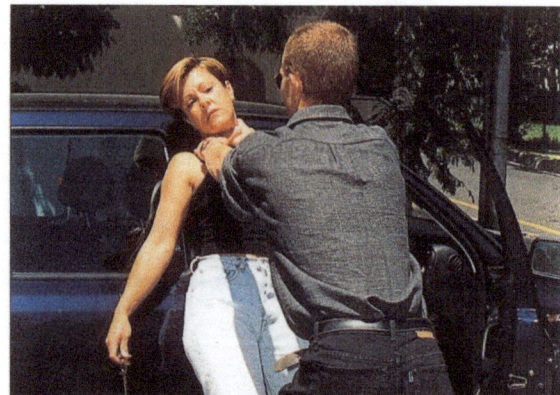

4 Hold onto your assailant's clothing to help you execute your technique. This will also help you establish better balance.

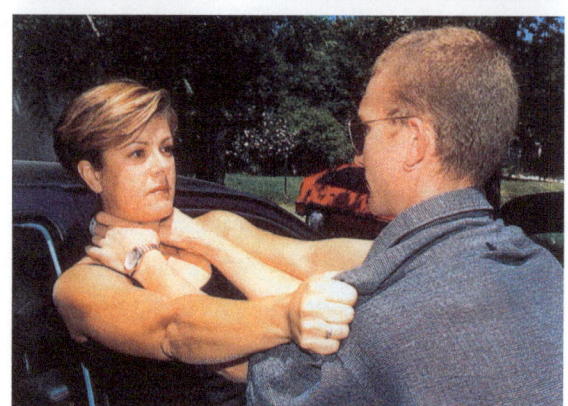

5 Your assailant is very close to you – a distance that is ideal for a knee technique to the groin. Do not release your grip on his clothing. Lift your knee up hard and fast between his legs, making sure to connect with his groin.

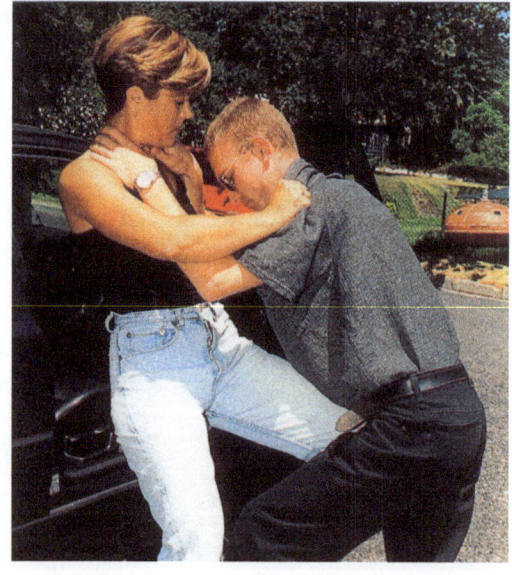

SELF-DEFENCE SCENARIOS

6 As your assailant folds over, follow up by jabbing your knee hard and fast onto his nose.

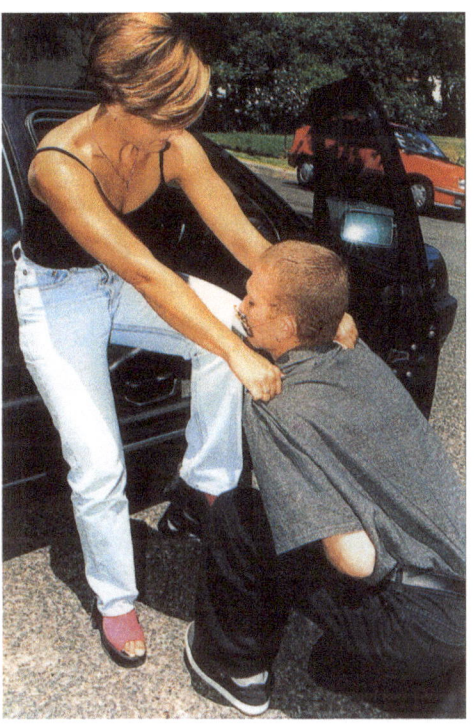

7 Push your assailant away from you. Either run to a group of people nearby or, if time permits, quickly get into your car and IMMEDIATELY lock the door.

◀ TIPS

» Although it may be difficult for you to breathe, DON'T PANIC.
» Do not fight power with power. In other words, do not waste valuable energy trying to pry his hands off your neck.
» Use your energy effectively by identifying an open target area on his body and applying an appropriate technique, in this instance, a knee to the groin. He is also wearing sunglasses. You could punch these hard into his face.

ATTACK TO THE THROAT WITH BOTH HANDS (2)

While bursting the eardrums has been featured as the first self-defence technique (Step 2), you could also poke his eyes, palm-heel strike your assailant's nose, strike or punch into his neck or Adam's apple, or use any combination of these.

1. Your assailant grabs your throat with both of his hands, pushing you up against a tree.

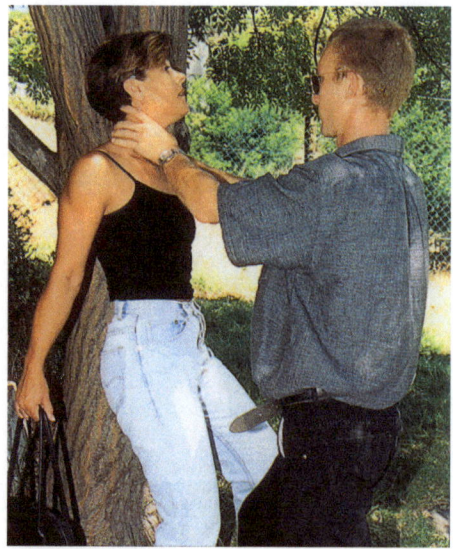

2. Use the tree to help you establish your balance. Cup both of your hands with your fingers together and wind up with your arms.

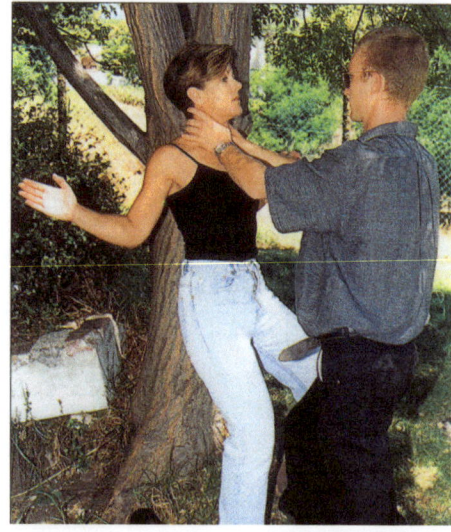

SELF-DEFENCE SCENARIOS

3 With a fast action (like playing the cymbals), hit your assailant's ears. Your point of contact should be the ears. This can cause the eardrums to burst.

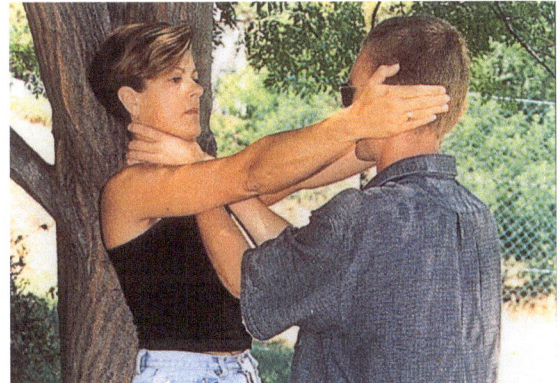

4 After you have completed the technique, pull your arms back towards your body for your follow-up technique.

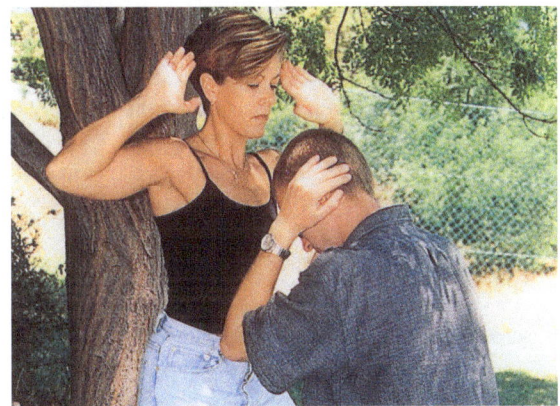

5 Your assailant has reacted by holding his hands to his ears, which makes the lower part of his body open for a follow-up technique. Turn your body slightly and perform the wind up for your next technique.

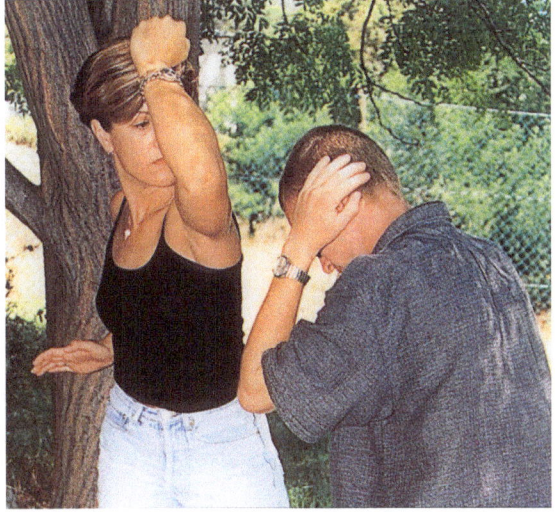

THE SOUTH AFRICAN WOMEN'S GUIDE TO SELF-DEFENCE

6 Shift your body as you feel necessary in order to get your hand or arm down for a strike to your assailant's groin.

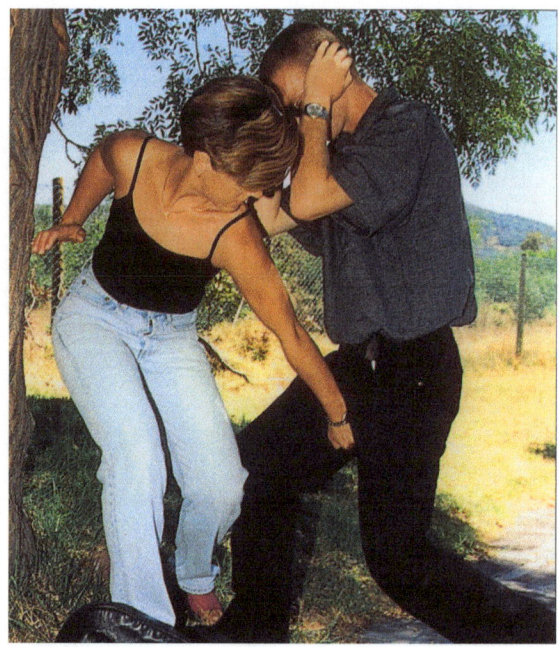

◀ TIPS

» Although it may be difficult for you to breathe, DON'T PANIC.
» Do not fight power with power. In other words, do not waste valuable energy trying to pry his hands off your neck.
» Use your energy effectively by identifying an open target area on his body and applying an appropriate technique. In this instance, his face and ears are initially the open targets.
» Use what you have near you to help you, for example, use the tree for balance. If his arms are too long and you cannot reach him, you will have to kick him first (see previous scenario, pages 97–99).

ATTACK TO THE THROAT WITH ONE HAND (1)

1. Your assailant grips your throat with one hand and pushes you up against a wall. With this one-hand grip, the thumb is the weak link. Turn your wrist to the outside and push a strong finger (or fingers) between your throat and his thumb. Grab onto his thumb with commitment.

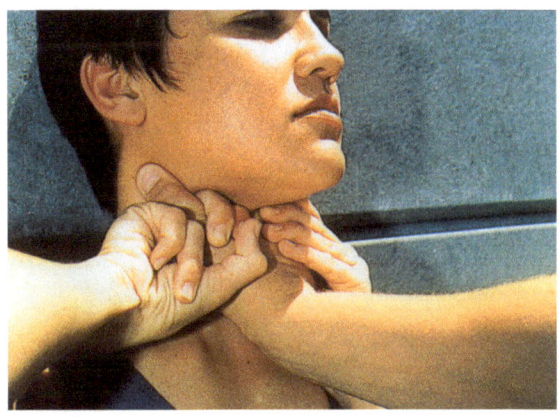

2. While your one hand is gripping his thumb, grab hold of the side of his hand with your other hand.

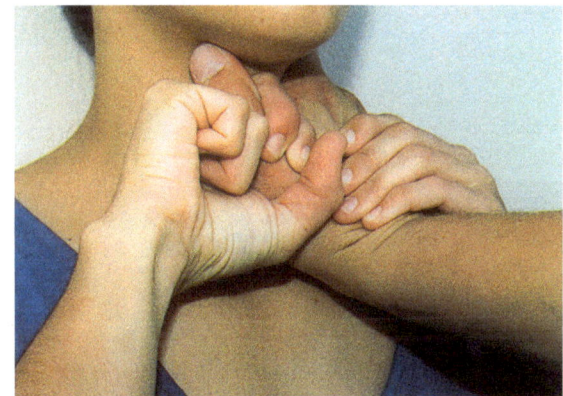

3. Turn both hands in a clockwise direction.

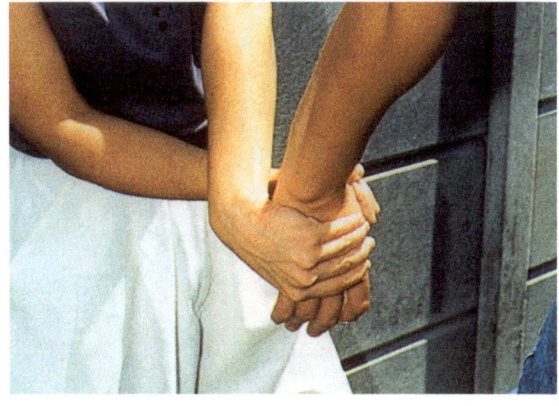

THE SOUTH AFRICAN WOMEN'S GUIDE TO SELF-DEFENCE

4 This motion forces your assailant to turn away from you (unless he is willing to snap his arm!). Maintain a strong hold of both his thumb and his hand.

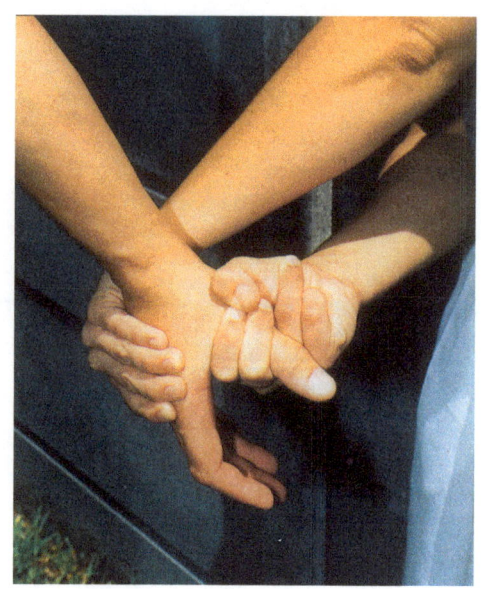

5 Kick with the side of your foot down onto the back of his leg/knee.

6 Wind up quickly with your elbow.

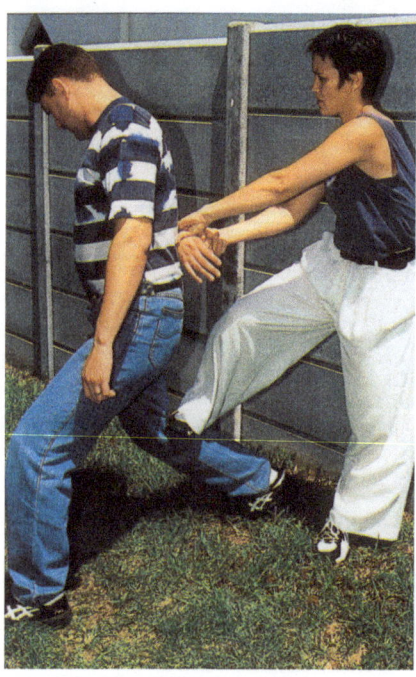

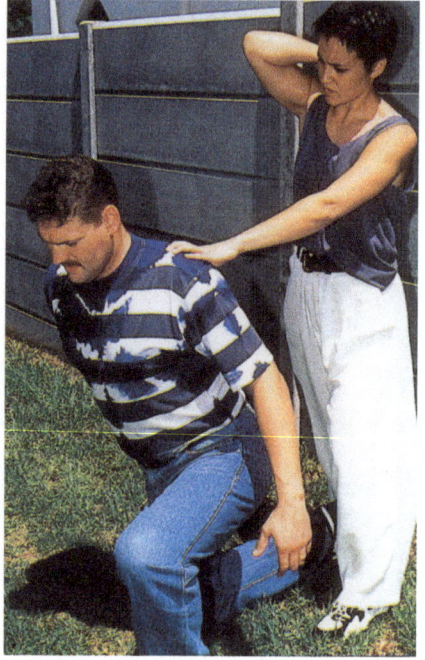

SELF-DEFENCE SCENARIOS

7 Strike down hard with your elbow onto the back of his neck between his shoulder blades.

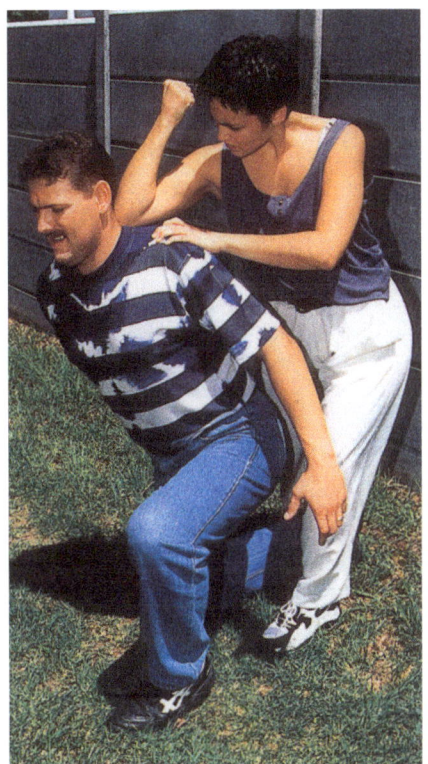

◀ TIPS

» The flesh on your neck is very pliable and loose. So is the piece of skin between your assailant's thumb and forefinger. Don't be afraid to really dig between your neck and this piece of skin to get a good hold of your assailant's thumb (even if it means that your fingernails cut into your skin).

» This technique will **not work** if your assailant has both hands around your neck and you try releasing both of his hands with both of yours.

ATTACK TO THE THROAT WITH ONE HAND (2)

1 Your assailant is strangling you with one hand around your throat.

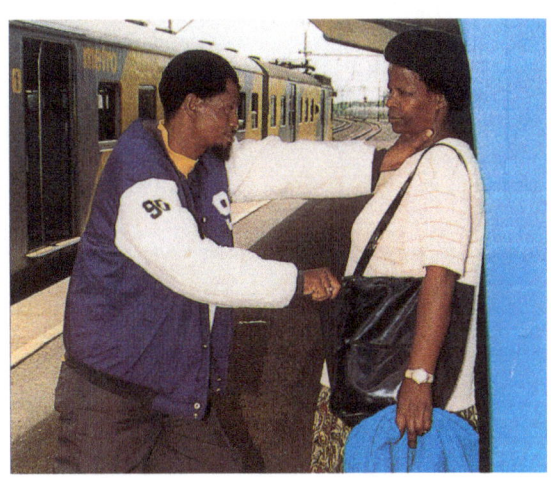

THE SOUTH AFRICAN WOMEN'S GUIDE TO SELF-DEFENCE

2. Lift up your arm and point your fingers (keeping them tightly together) towards his throat.

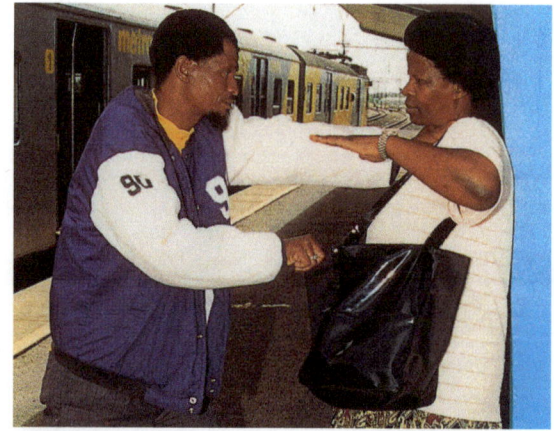

3. Spear strike with the point of your fingers into your assailant's throat (see Basic Self-Defence Techniques, page 86).

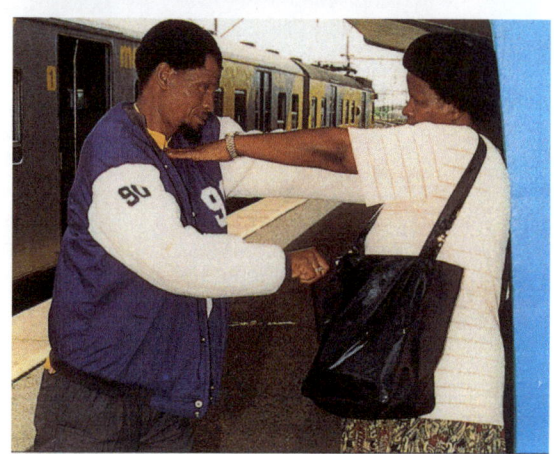

4. Your assailant will release his grip on your throat.

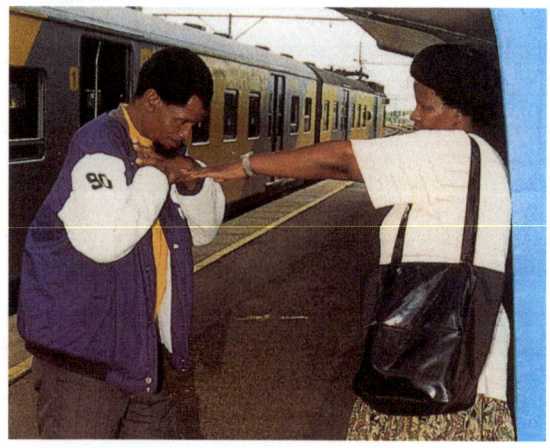

SELF-DEFENCE SCENARIOS

5 Follow up your defence by swinging your leg up between his legs (as high as you can), while holding onto his clothing for balance.

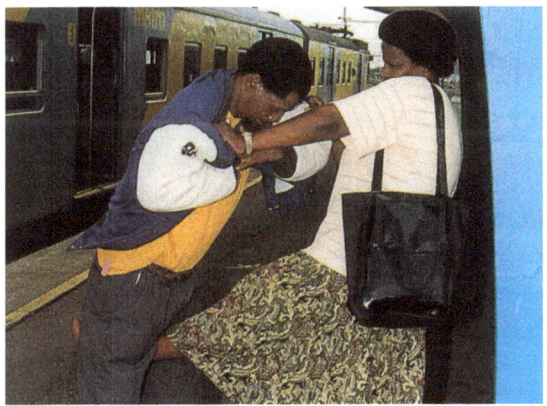

◀ TIPS

» As an alternative to the first technique, you could throw your jersey into your attacker's face to distract him or obscure his vision and then use this opportunity to apply your techniques.
» Other techniques you can use instead of the spear strike are a hard punch to his nose or a finger-poke to his eyes, or these can be used as follow-up techniques. There are no limits to the number of techniques you may apply.

ATTACK TO THE THROAT WITH ONE HAND (3)

1 Your assailant is gripping your throat with one hand and pushing you up against a wall.

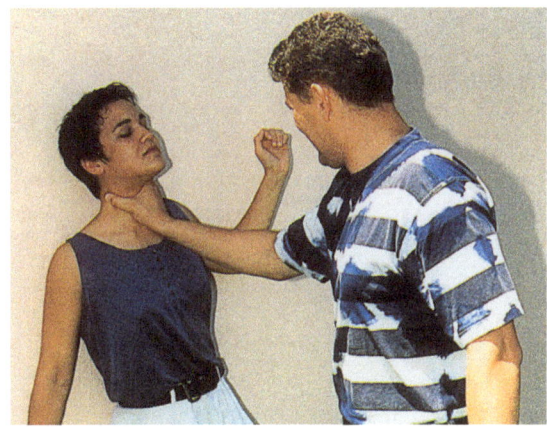

2. Take two of your strong fingers, squeeze them in between your throat and his thumb, and grab tightly onto his thumb.

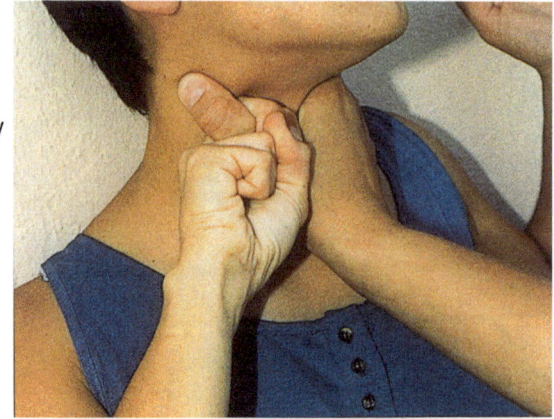

3. Turn his thumb backwards.

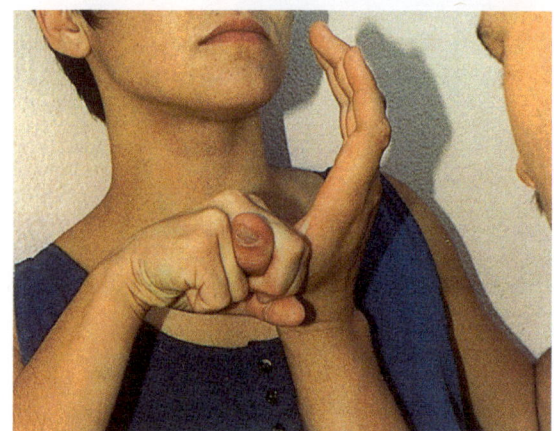

4. Whilst turning his thumb backwards, place your other hand on his elbow.

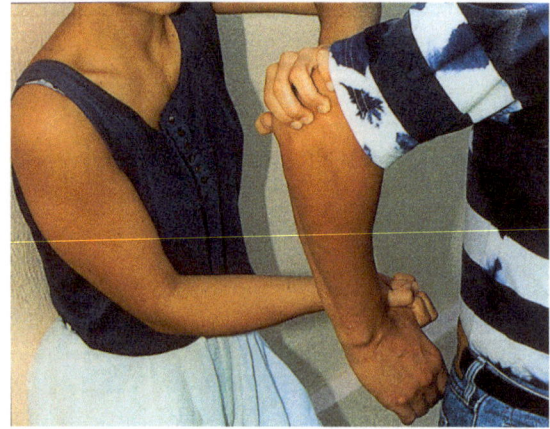

5 Twist his arm in a clockwise direction.

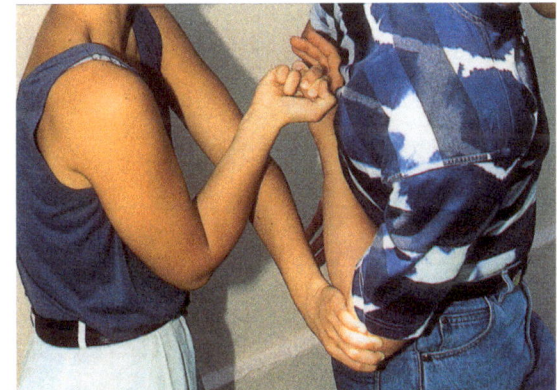

6 While still holding his elbow in position, wind up high with your other arm.

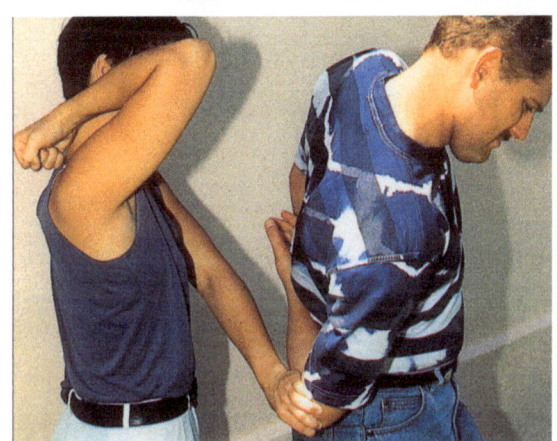

7 Strike down hard with your elbow between his shoulder blades.

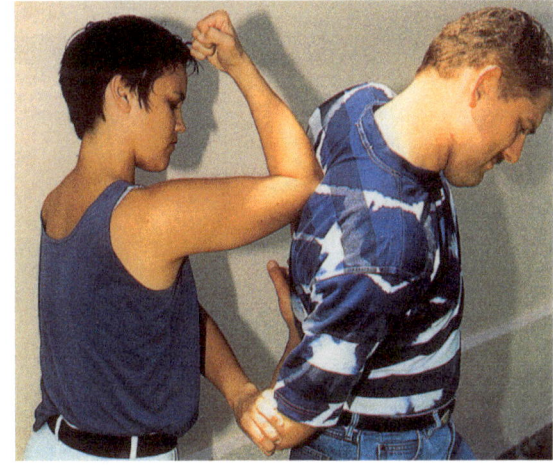

THE SOUTH AFRICAN WOMEN'S GUIDE TO SELF-DEFENCE

8 Push your assailant away and remove yourself from the situation.

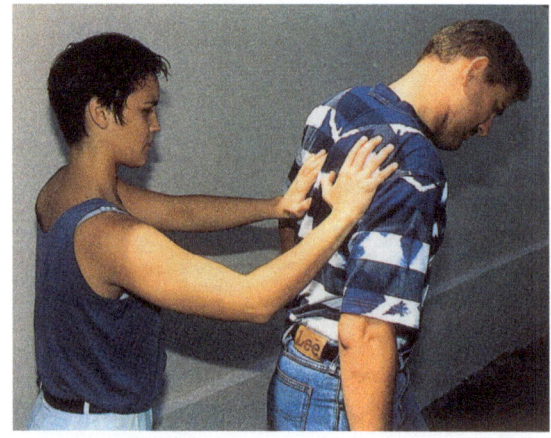

WRIST GRAB WITH ONE HAND (1)

1 Your assailant grabs your wrist.

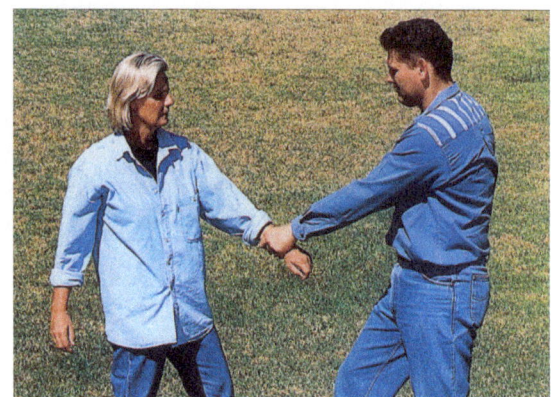

2 Wind up with your other hand and make a fist. At the same time, slightly raise the middle (strong) knuckle of the fist that is winding up (see Basic Self-Defence Techniques, page 92).

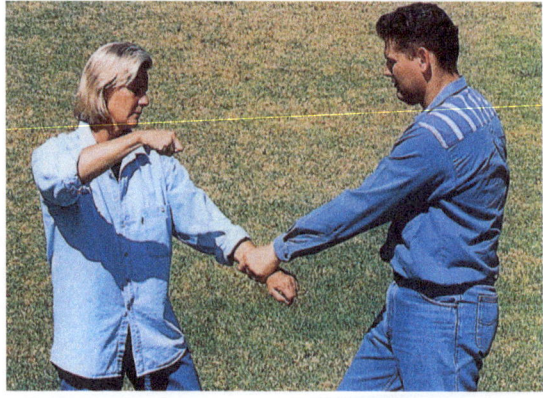

SELF-DEFENCE SCENARIOS

3 Hit down hard with your raised knuckle on the back of your assailant's hand.

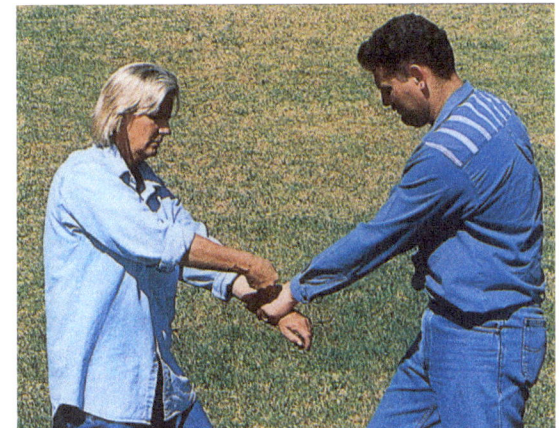

4 Bring the same arm back (wind up) and make a fist.

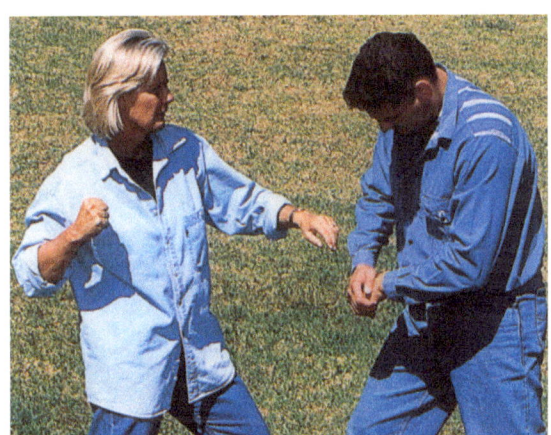

5 Hit your assailant hard on the nose.

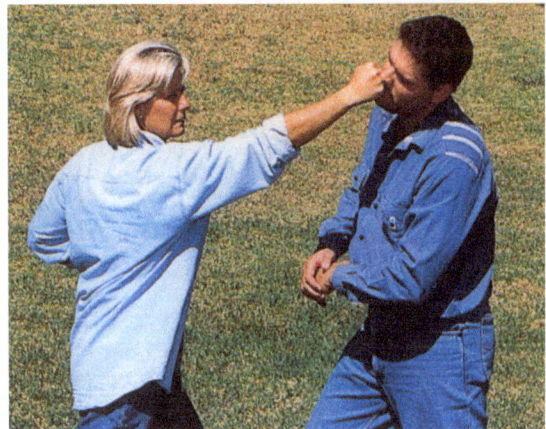

THE SOUTH AFRICAN WOMEN'S GUIDE TO SELF-DEFENCE

6 Follow up by swinging your leg up between your assailant's legs.

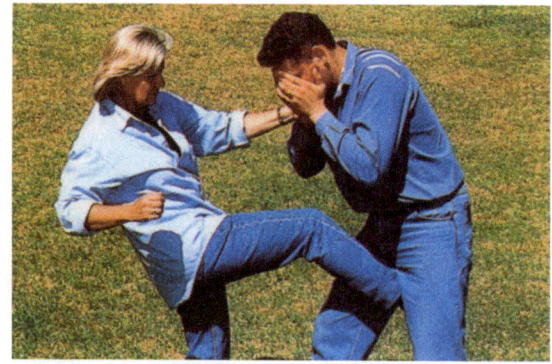

7 Wind up high with your arm.

8 Bring your elbow down hard onto the back of your assailant's neck or between his shoulder blades.

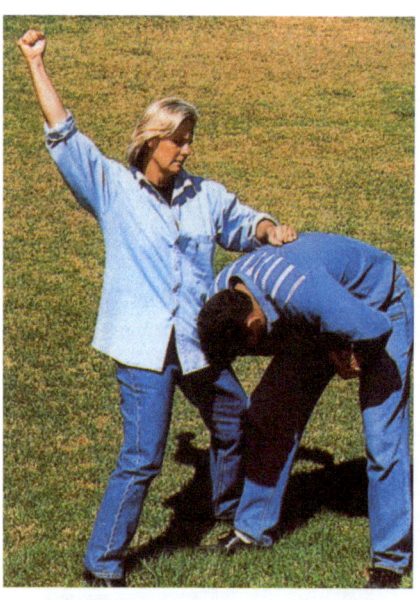

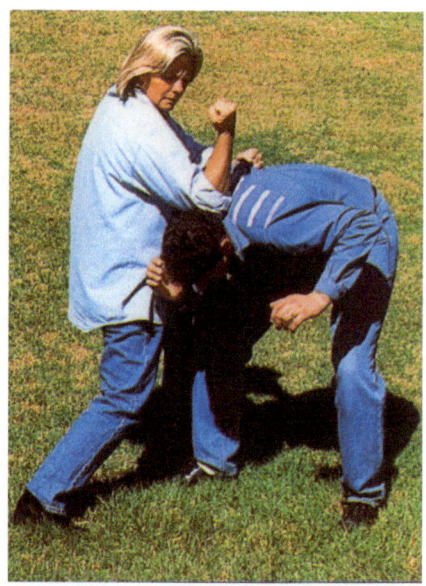

◀ TIPS

» This technique is usually used when the assailant grabs you with the same arm (his left arm grabs your left arm), but can also be used if he grabs you with his opposite hand (your left wrist with his right hand).

SELF-DEFENCE SCENARIOS

WRIST-GRAB WITH ONE HAND (2)

1. Your assailant grabs your arm (opposite arm to his).

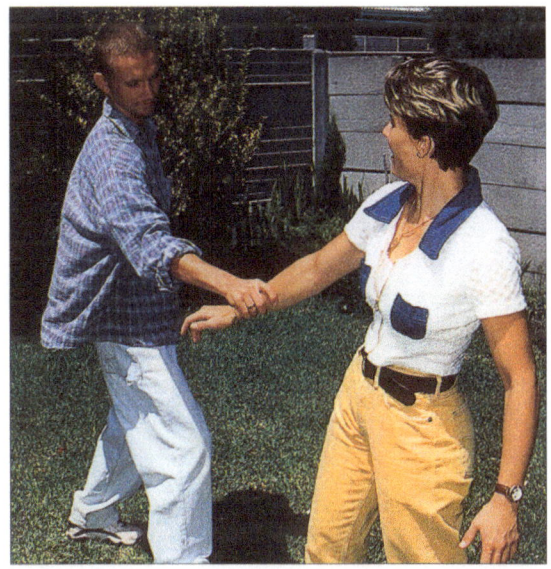

2. As he grabs your arm, twist your hand slightly and grab onto his arm.

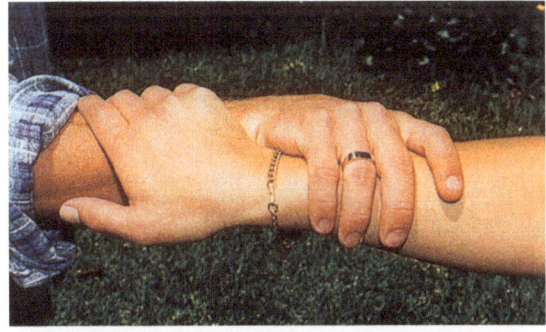

3. Quickly place your other hand on top of your assailant's hand.

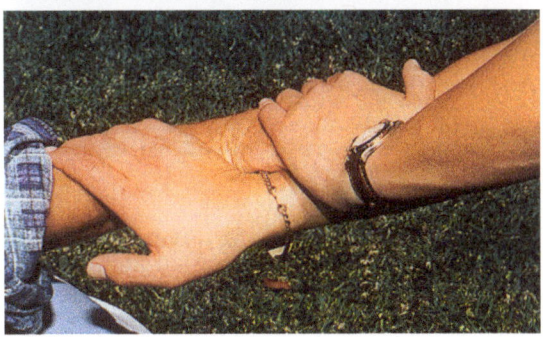

113

THE SOUTH AFRICAN WOMEN'S GUIDE TO SELF-DEFENCE

4 Forcefully push both your hands downwards (towards the ground) and towards you. This will force your assailant to his knees.

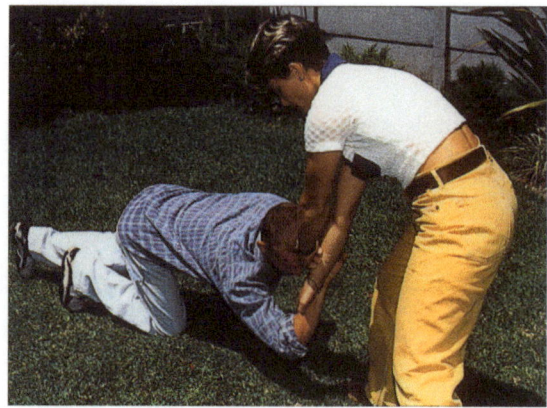

5 Wind up high with your heel.

6 Kick down hard onto the back of your assailant's neck.

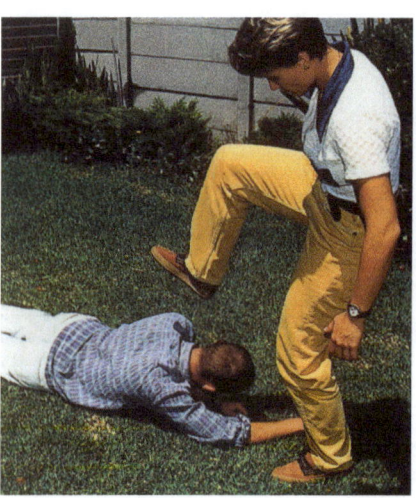
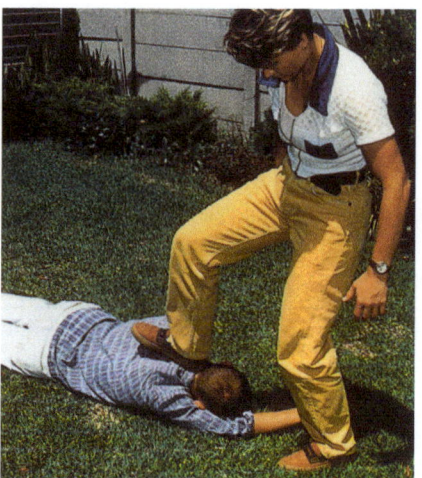

◀ **TIPS**

» When pushing your hands downwards and towards you, **do not** lower your body as you do so. Keep your arms and back as straight as possible. Concentrate on pulling your arms down towards your groin area.
» This can be a difficult technique if your assailant's arms are too wide for you to get a reasonable grip, or if he has grabbed you directly ON your wrist. If this is the case, use the techniques in variation 1 on pages 110–112.

SELF-DEFENCE SCENARIOS

GENERAL ATTACKS TO THE FACE

1. The assailant attempts to strike your face with his hand.

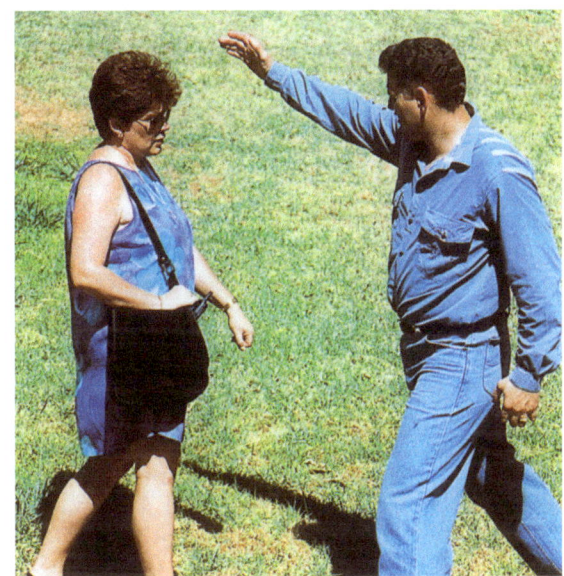

2. Block his strike with your arm by lifting your elbow up high (see Basic blocking, page 79).

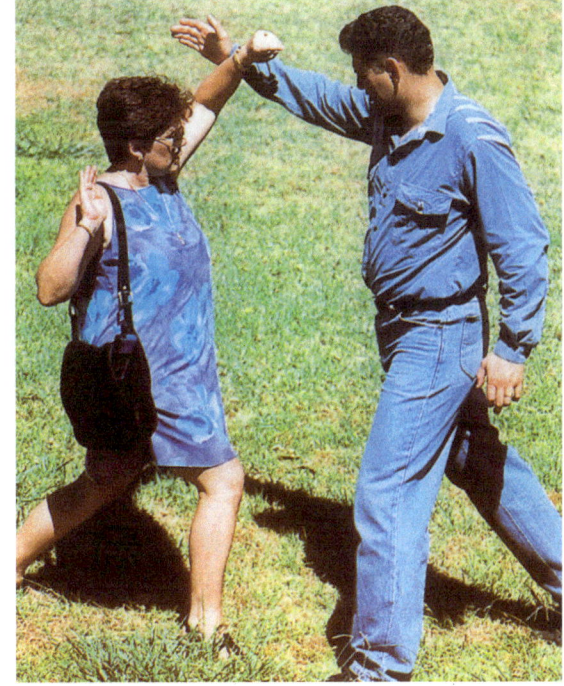

3 Using the palm-heel of your hand, hit your assailant hard on his nose. (Pull your fingers back when doing this technique.)

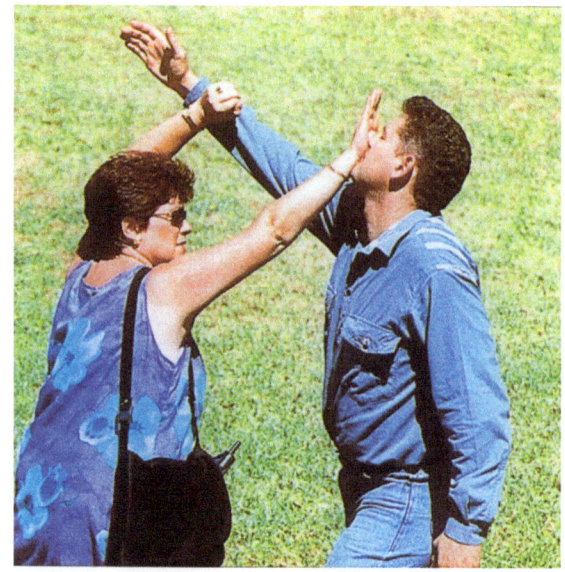

4 Swing your leg up and hard between the assailant's legs.

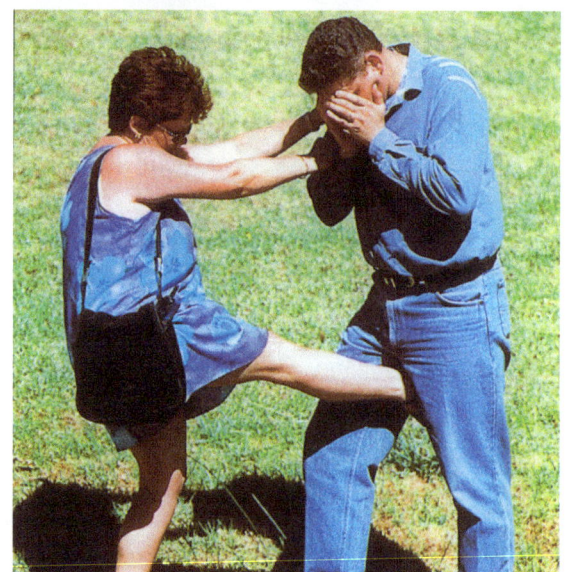

◀ TIPS

» The upward block (step 2) must be done very quickly.
» An alternative to the upward block would be a body shift, for example backwards, away from the attacker, or to the left or right.

SELF-DEFENCE SCENARIOS

GENERAL ATTACK FROM THE FRONT

Many women are attacked in their homes. A house is full of potential weapons, so before discarding anything you may be holding onto at the time of the attack, first assess whether it will be useful to you as a weapon. If you can use it, do so. It may be a hot iron, kitchen knife, vacuum nozzle (jab), aerosol can (spray), or a broom.

1. Your assailant approaches you. Use whatever you have in your hands to defend yourself, or pick up something nearby to assist you, for example a vase, an ashtray, scissors, etc.

2. In this case, you have a broom. Turn the broomstick so that the handle points towards your assailant.

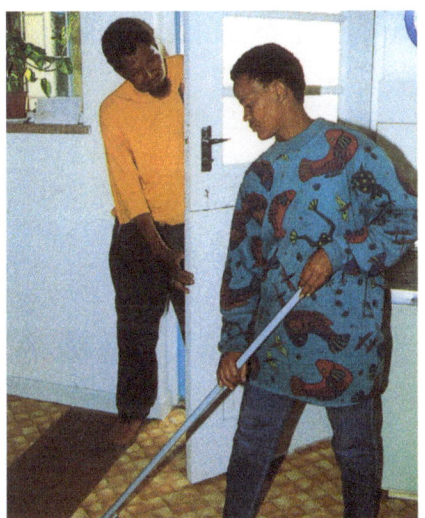

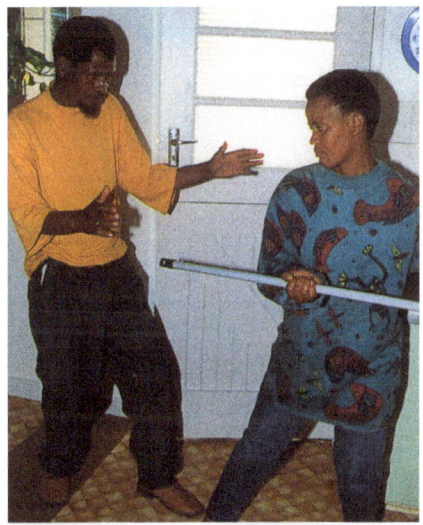

3. Jab the broomstick as hard as you can into the assailant's stomach.

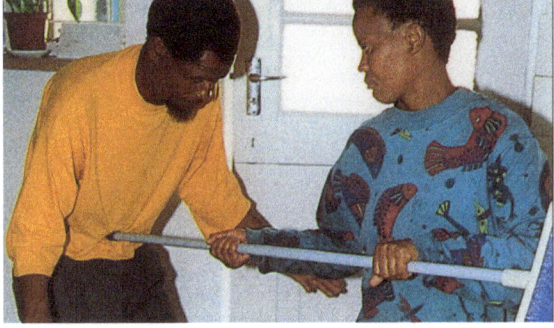

THE SOUTH AFRICAN WOMEN'S GUIDE TO SELF-DEFENCE

4 Wind up to gain momentum.

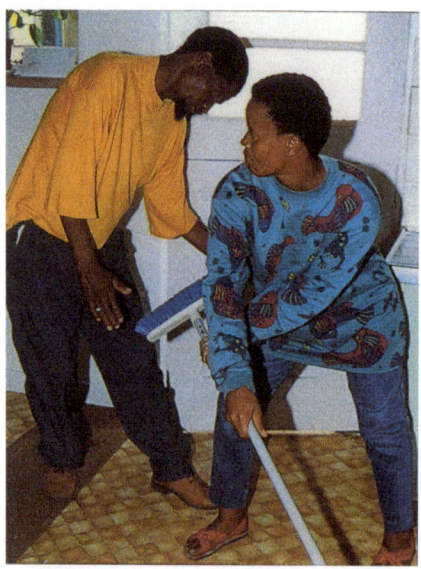

5 Strike the side of the assailant's neck with the handle of the broomstick.

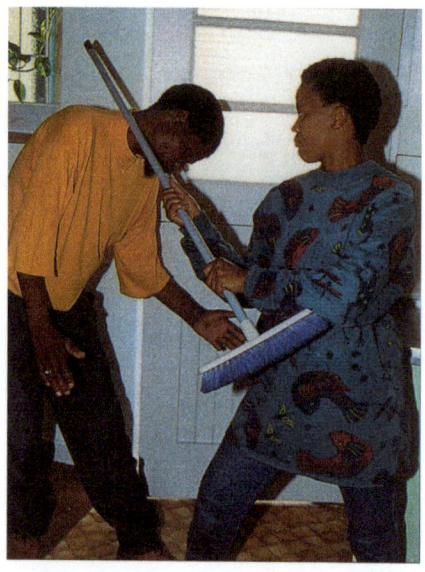

6 Pull the broomstick back and wind up.

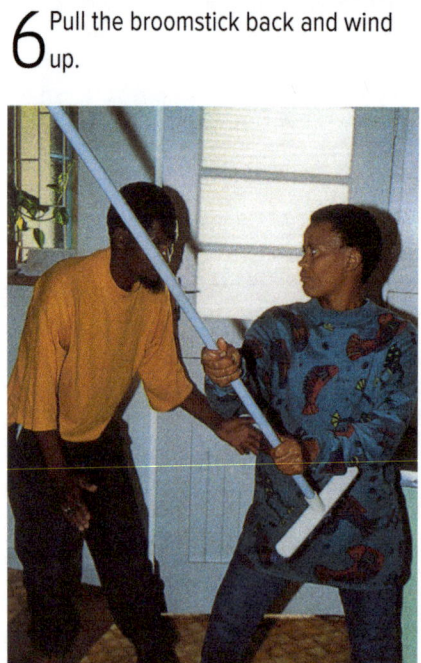

7 Strike it down hard onto his knee.

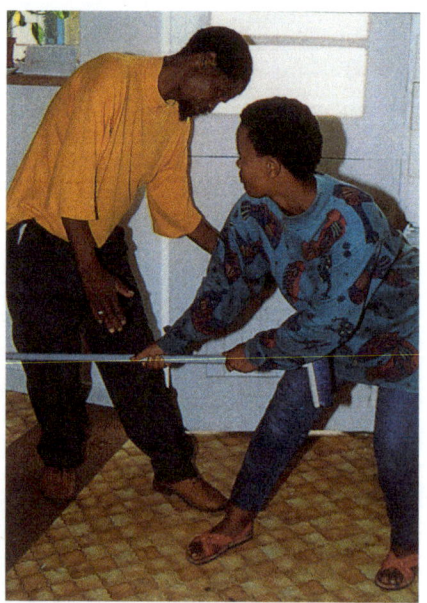

SELF-DEFENCE SCENARIOS

8 Pull the broomstick back and wind up again for momentum.

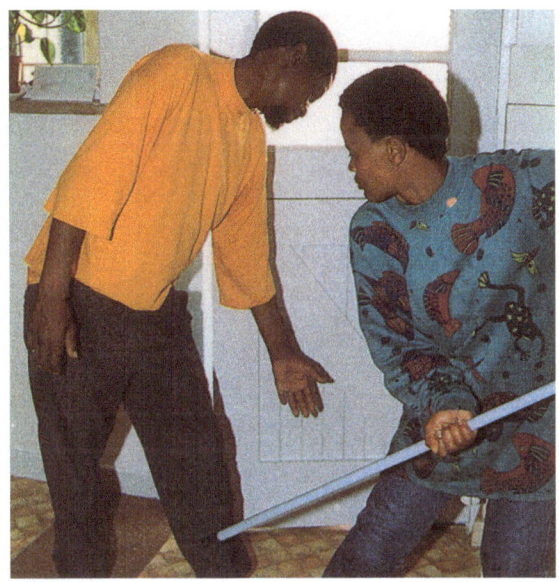

9 Hit up between the assailant's legs into his groin.

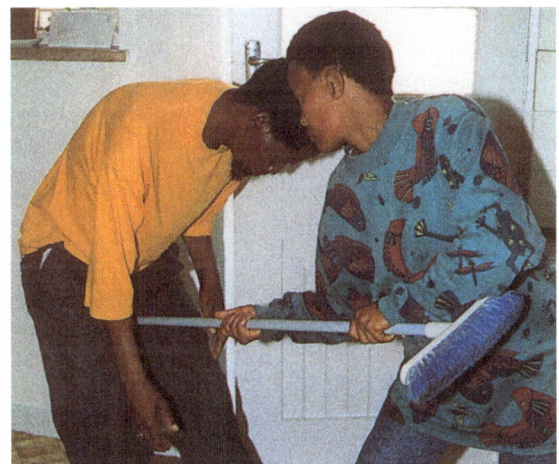

◀ TIPS

» If you do not have enough space to wind up with the broom (step 4), just keep jabbing it (step 3) into his body target areas, such as face, throat, groin, and the front of his body.

ATTACKS FROM BEHIND

ATTACK FROM BEHIND WITH ONE ARM AROUND THE THROAT

1. Your assailant strangles you from behind with one arm around your throat.

2. Wind up with your hand and arm.

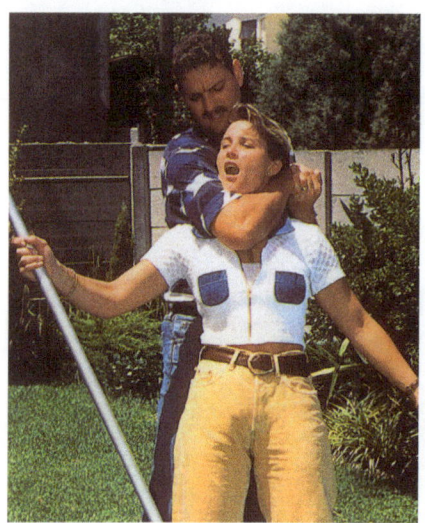
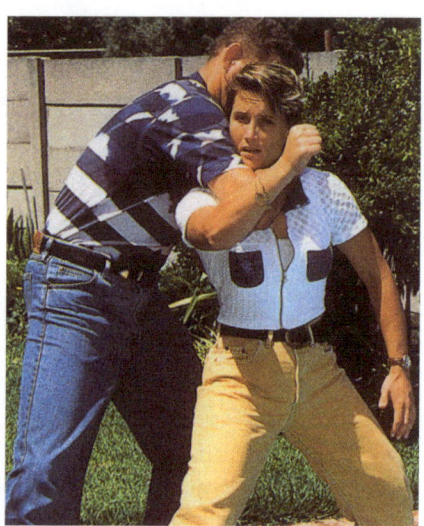

3. Shift your hip to the side and strike down hard into his groin with your hand.

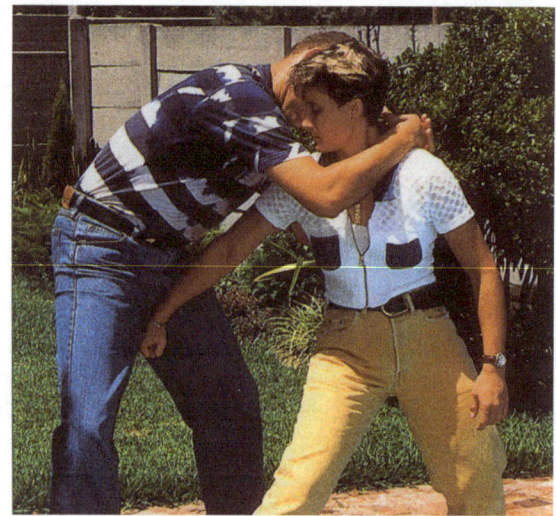

SELF-DEFENCE SCENARIOS

4 Move your body to the side and wind up with both hands clenched together.

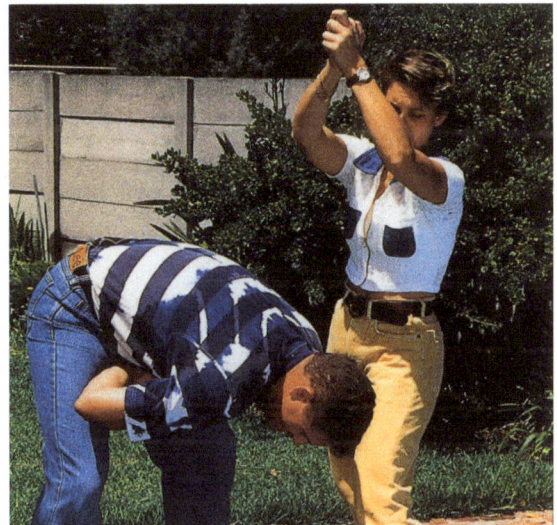

5 Hit down hard onto the back of your assailant's neck with your clenched hands. You can also bring your elbow down hard onto the back of his neck or between his shoulder blades.

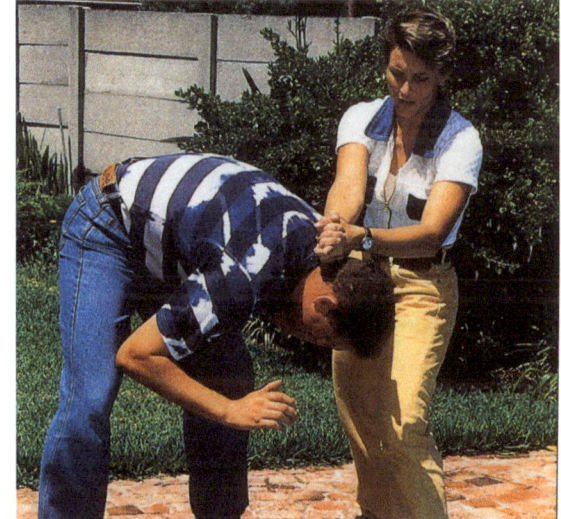

◀ **TIPS**

» The strike down to your assailant's groin (step 3) can be made with a closed fist or the outer edge of an open hand (see Basic Self-Defence Techniques, page 89).

THE SOUTH AFRICAN WOMEN'S GUIDE TO SELF-DEFENCE

BEAR-HUG (1)

1. Your assailant approaches you from behind, grabs you in a bear-hug grip and lifts you off your feet. Hang like a dead weight.

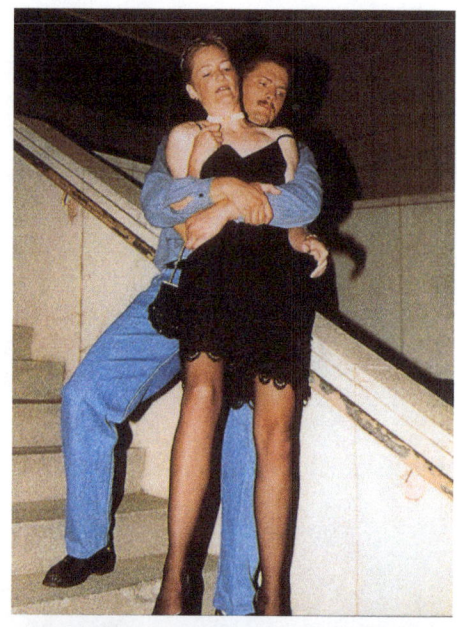

2. Wait until the assailant puts you down and establish your balance as quickly as possible.

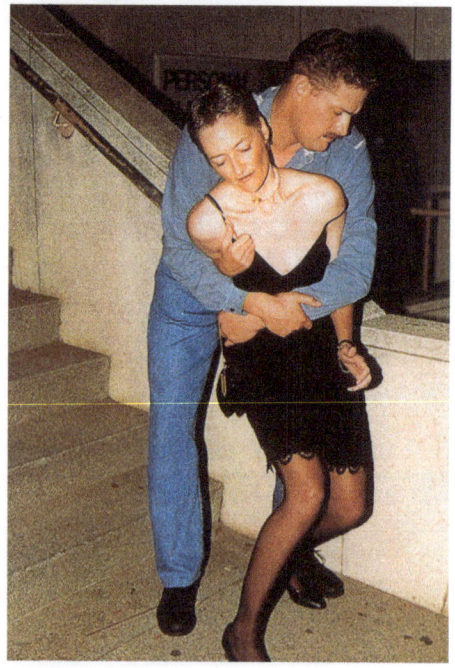

SELF-DEFENCE SCENARIOS

3 Look down to see where the assailant has placed his feet. Lift your knee up high as a wind up for your next technique.

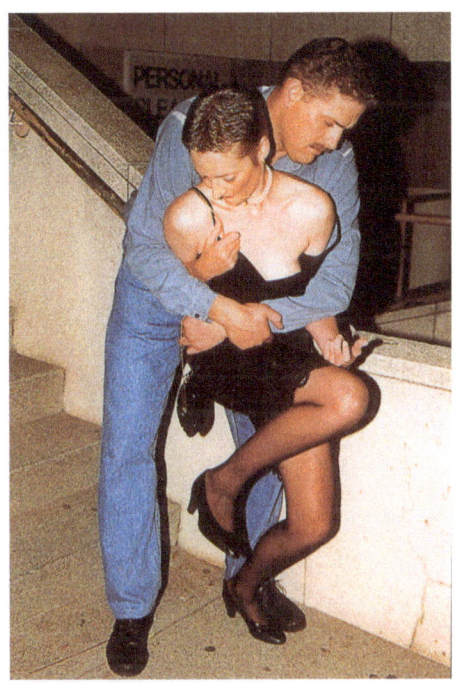

4 Stamp down hard onto your assailant's foot (the closest and most accessible one) with the heel of your shoe.

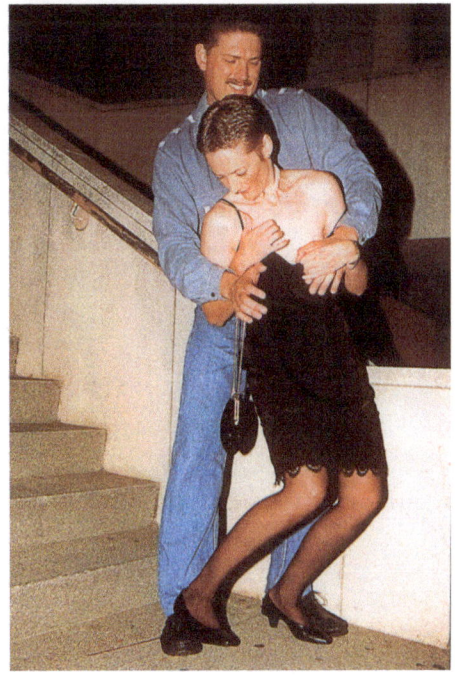

5 Move your body out of your assailant's grip, grab hold of his hair (or ears or head) and bring your knee up hard onto his nose.

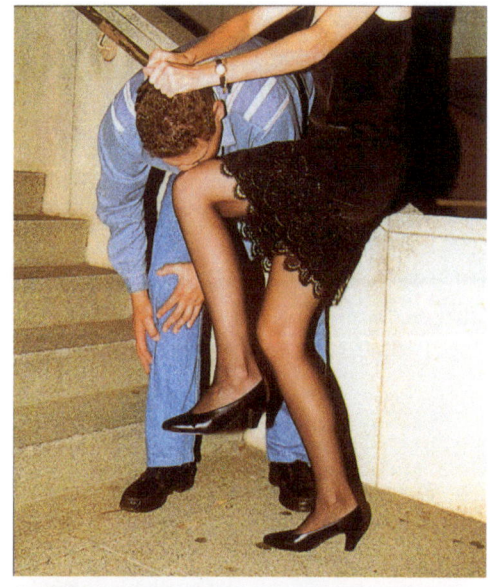

6 Push the assailant away.

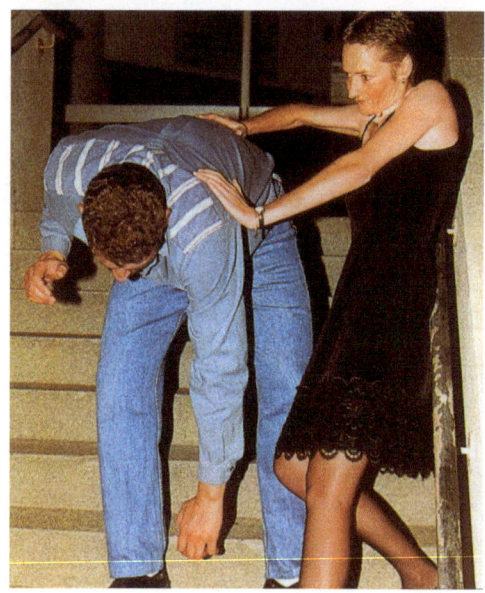

◀ TIPS

» After pushing your assailant away, don't immediately turn your back on him. Keep an eye on him until you have retreated a reasonable distance.

BEAR-HUG (2)

1. Your assailant grabs both your arms from behind with a bear-hug grip. Look quickly to see where his feet are placed. Lift your knee up high as a wind up for your next technique.

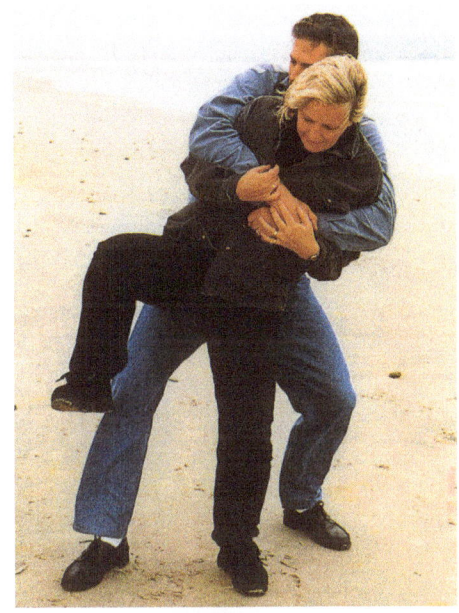

2. Stamp down hard with the heel of your foot onto your assailant's foot. His grip should loosen slightly.

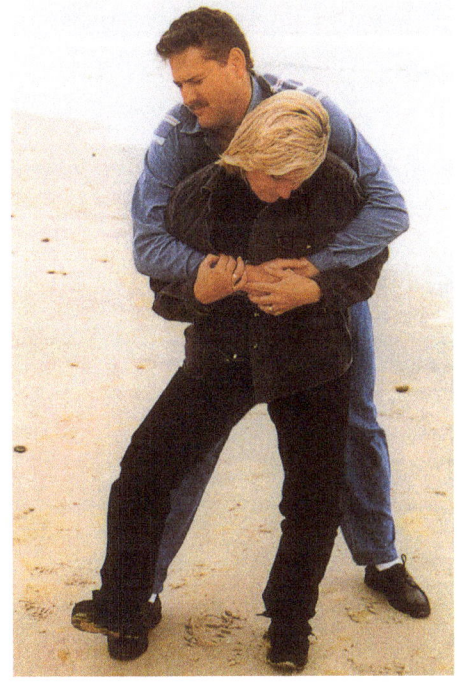

THE SOUTH AFRICAN WOMEN'S GUIDE TO SELF-DEFENCE

3 Drop your hipline down by moving your legs into a wide, firm stance, and blocking upwards with both your arms. This must be done quickly, and preferably in one movement.

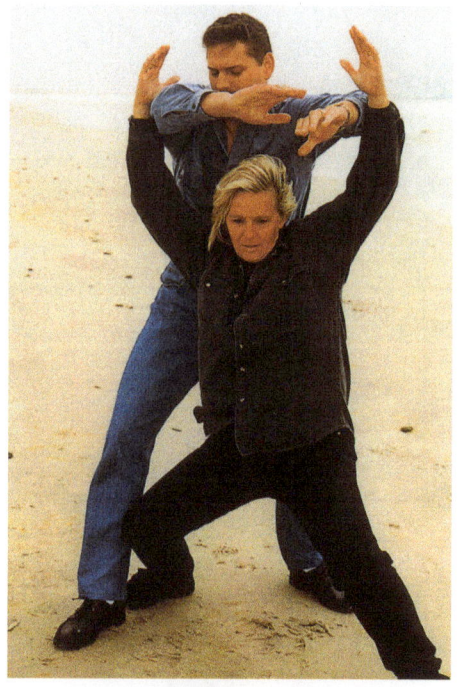

4 Wind up with your elbow and identify the available target areas.

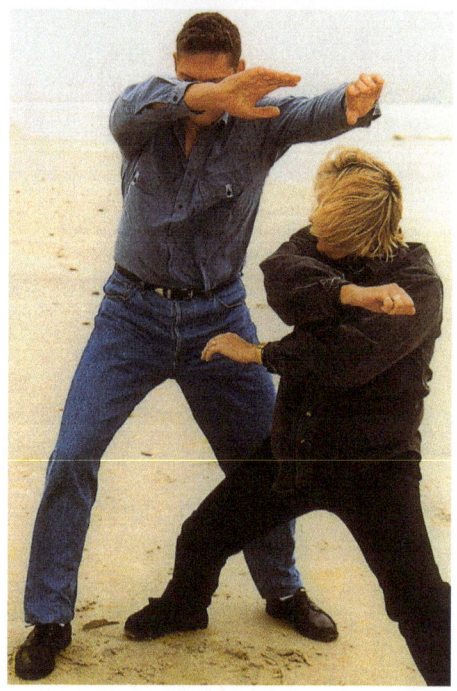

SELF-DEFENCE SCENARIOS

5 Hit your attacker's body hard with your elbow. Repeat the elbow strike at least three times, winding up with your elbow each time to ensure a full blow.

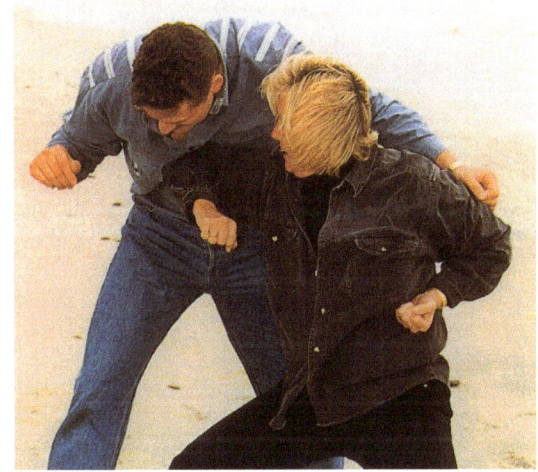

6 Push your assailant away and remove yourself from the situation.

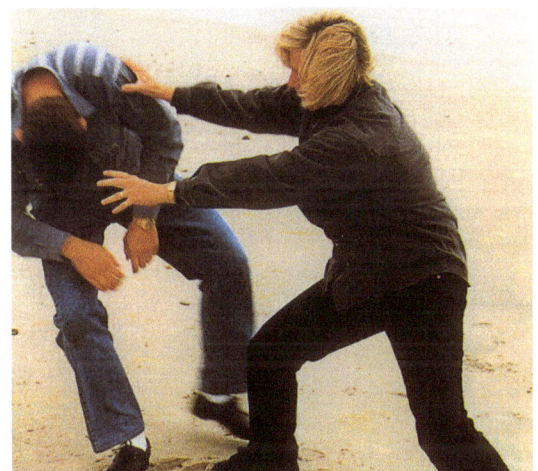

◀ TIPS

» A good, strong elbow technique is effective on any part of a man's body. A punch, however, is not. Punches should only be directed to the face, chin, neck, solar plexus, groin and throat. Because the solar plexus is a relatively small area, it is also recommended that you don't punch there unless you are quite familiar with its location.

MOUTH AND WAIST GRIP

1. Your assailant approaches you from behind. He covers your mouth with one hand and grabs you around your body with his other arm.

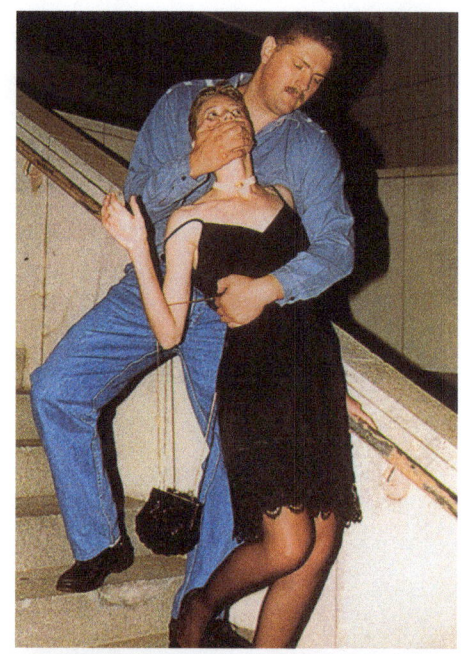

2. Wind up with your free hand and arm. If you feel unbalanced or uncomfortable on the stairs, hold onto the stair rail to assist your balance.

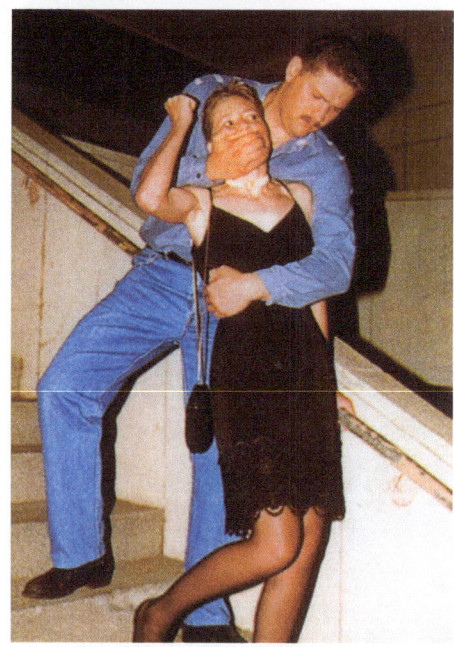

3 Shift your hip to the side and hit downward with your arm into your assailant's groin.

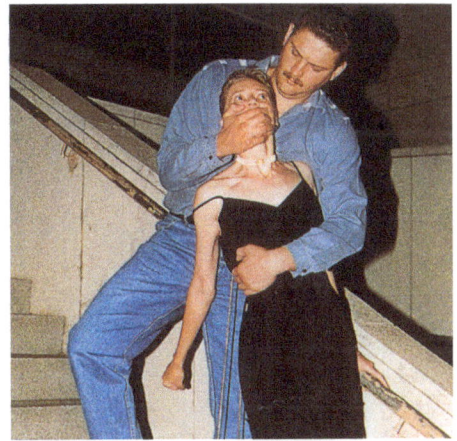

4 Lift up the same arm and grab your assailant's hair.

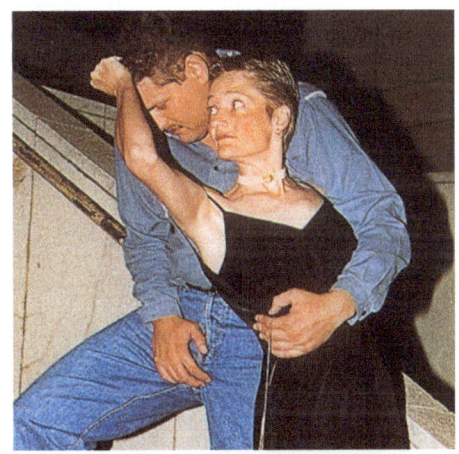

5 Using your grip on his hair, pull his head over your shoulder while shifting your body further to the side.

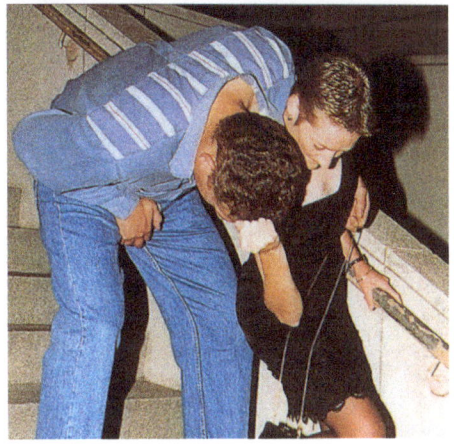

THE SOUTH AFRICAN WOMEN'S GUIDE TO SELF-DEFENCE

6 Still holding his hair, bring your knee up high for the wind up to your next technique.

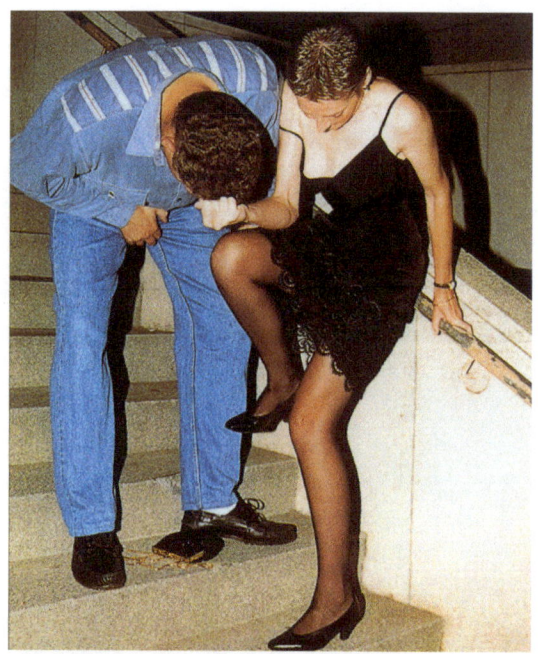

7 Kick down hard onto his foot with the heel of your shoe.

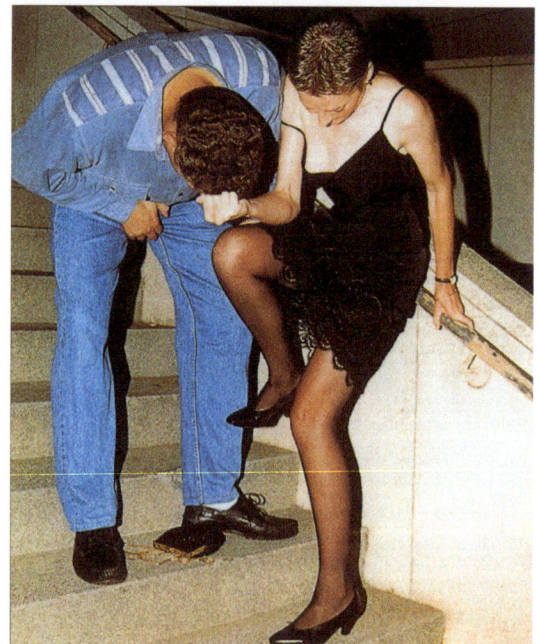

SELF-DEFENCE SCENARIOS

8 Wind up high with your elbow

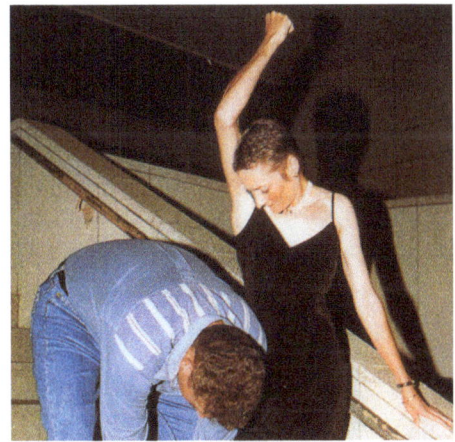

9 Strike down hard with your elbow between his shoulder blades or onto the back of his neck.

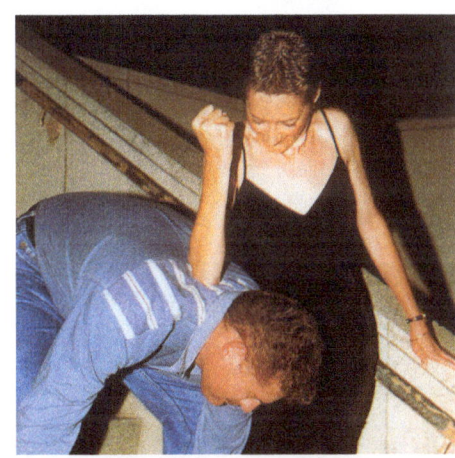

10 Push him away from you and remove yourself from the situation.

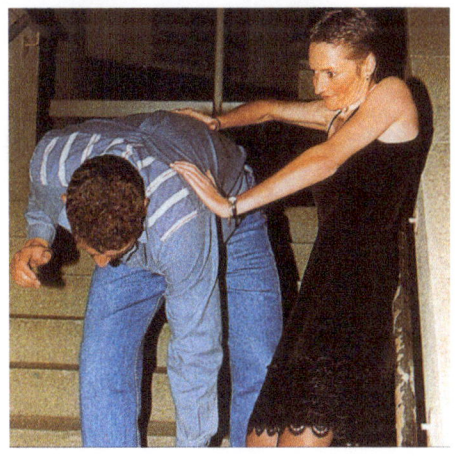

ARMLOCK ATTACK WITH BOTH HANDS

1. Your assailant grabs your arm and forces it into an armlock position behind your back.

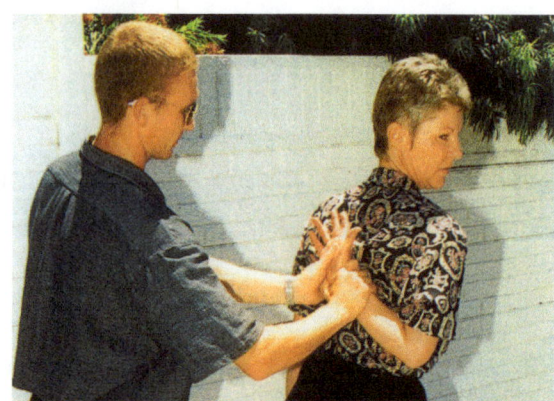

2. Take a big step forward, lowering your upper body slightly as you do so to release the pressure from the armlock and straighten your arm.

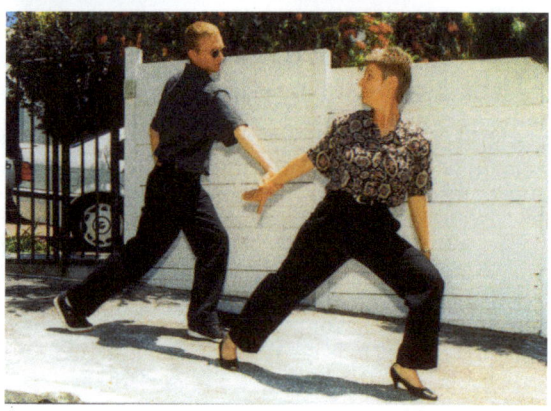

3. Grab your assailant's wrist as you turn your body.

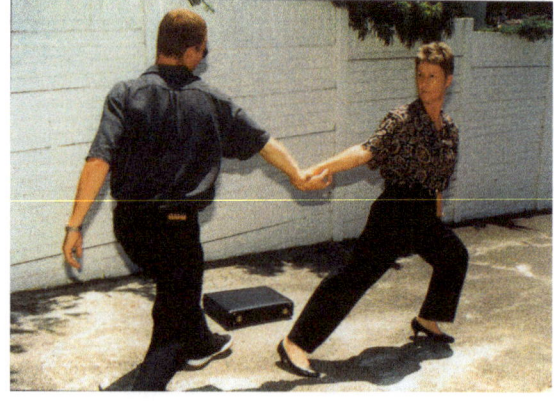

SELF-DEFENCE SCENARIOS

4 Complete the turn until you are facing him and hold onto his wrist with your other hand for balance.

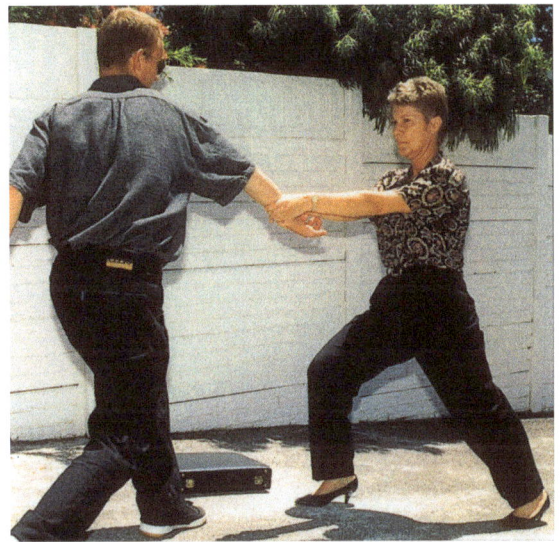

5 Swing your leg up and kick between your assailant's legs, into his groin.

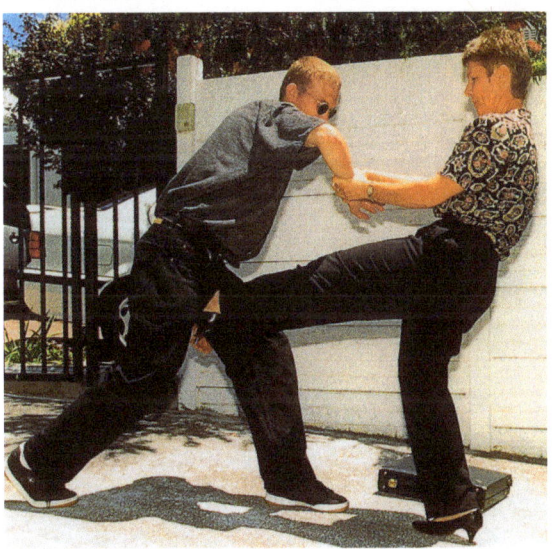

◀ TIPS

» It is very important to bend your body forwards and down as you move away (step 2), otherwise the grip on your arm will be very painful.

HAIR GRAB FROM BEHIND

1. Your assailant grabs your hair from behind with one hand and pulls you down onto the ground.

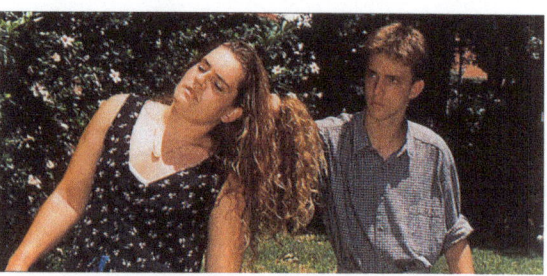

2. He places both of his hands around your throat.

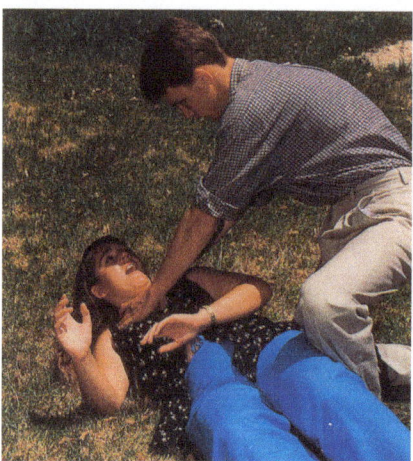

3. He attempts to climb on top of you. His arms could be in the way, making it difficult for you to punch his nose. The open and accessible target area here is his groin. Strike into his groin with your open hand, and then pull.

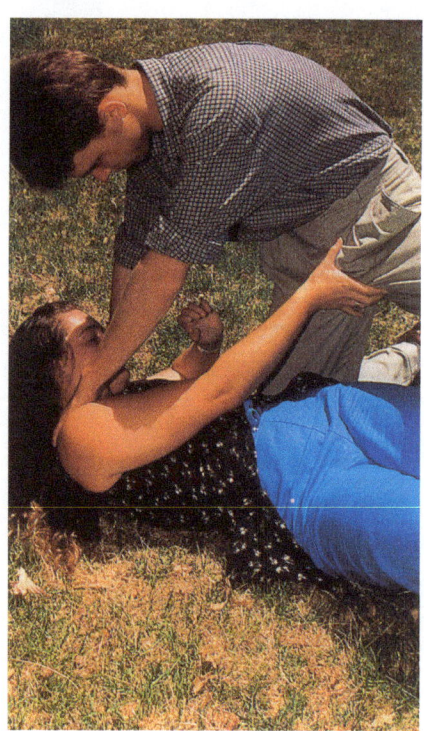

◀ TIPS

» Don't try to pry his hands away from your neck – you'll waste a lot of valuable energy.
» A strike to his groin is an effective technique here. A strike or punch to his face may have been difficult because of the position of his arms.

SELF-DEFENCE SCENARIOS

SINGLE-ARM GRIP AROUND THE THROAT

1. Your assailant grabs you from behind with one arm around your throat.

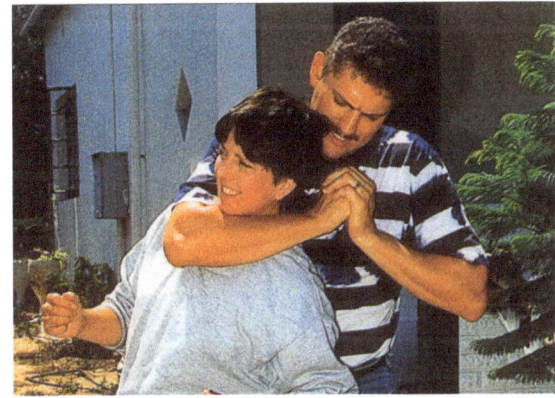

2. Lift your arm up high and grab his ear on the open side of his body.

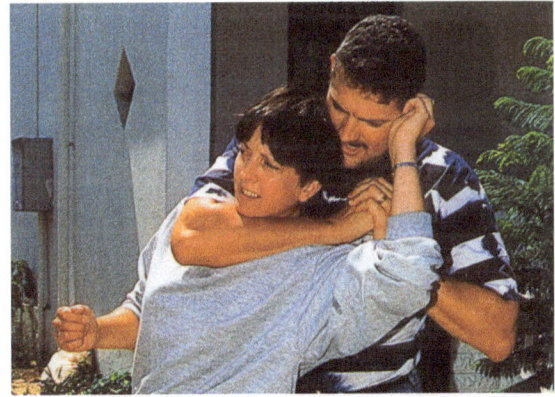

3. Keeping a tight grip on his ear, twist it and pull hard.

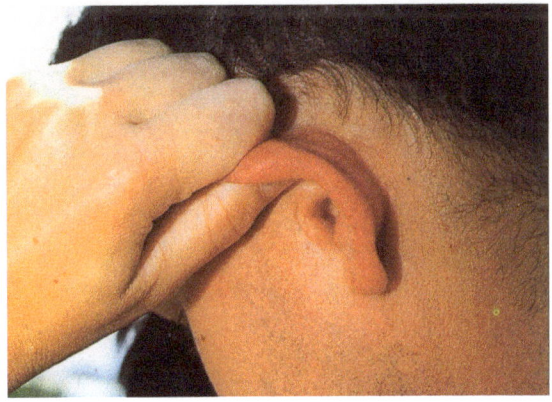

4. Keep pulling until you have forced his head over your shoulder. This should be done while moving your body to the side, until you are facing him.

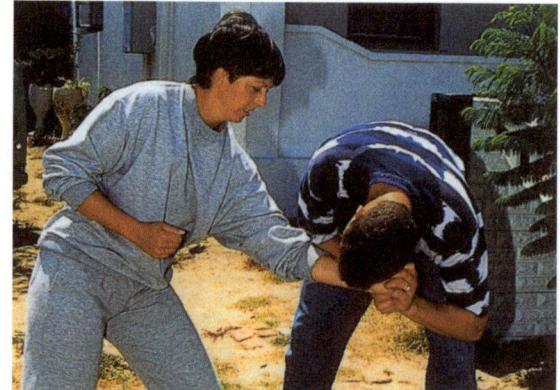

5. Release your grip on his ear. With one hand, grab hold of his shoulder or clothing for balance, and with the other, grab him behind his head. Bring your knee up in a hard strike to his nose.

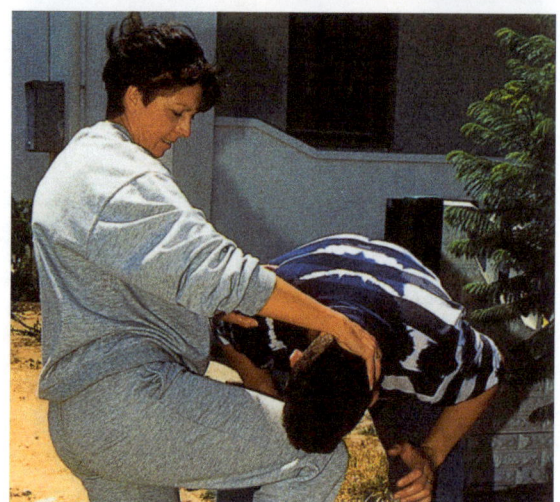

6. Put your foot down again for balance. Wind up with both arms and cup your hands, keeping your fingers together (see Basic Self-Defence Techniques, page 82).

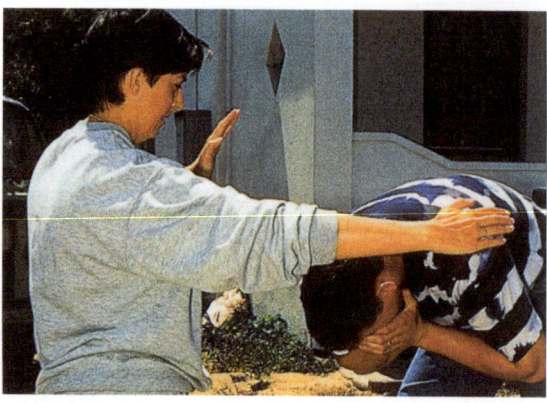

SELF-DEFENCE SCENARIOS

7 Hit his ears with your cupped hands (you could burst his eardrums).

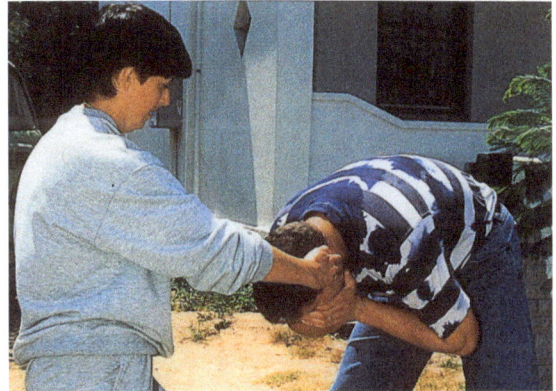

8 Grab onto your assailant for balance and swing your leg high between his legs, into his groin.

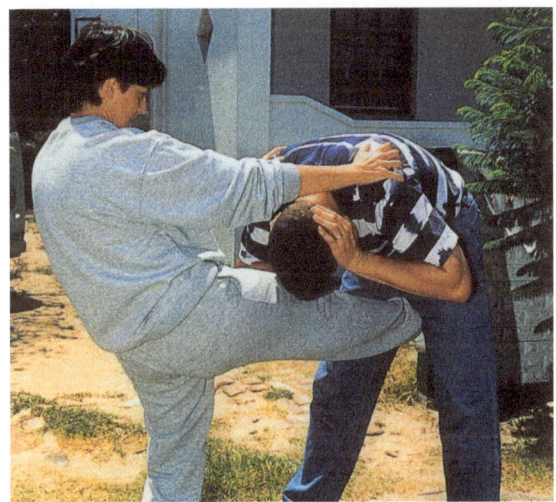

9 Push your assailant away and remove yourself from the situation.

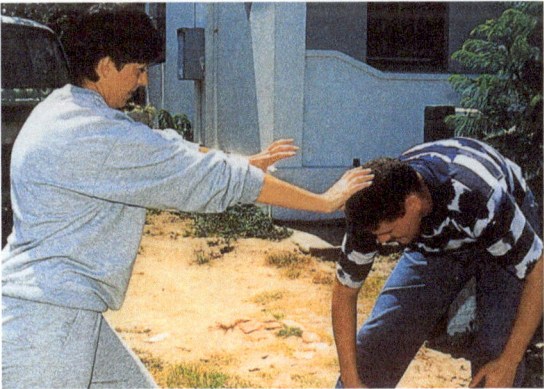

ATTACKS FROM THE SIDE

STRANGLEHOLD WITH ONE ARM AROUND THE NECK (1)

1. Your assailant grabs you around the neck with one arm and locks his hands.

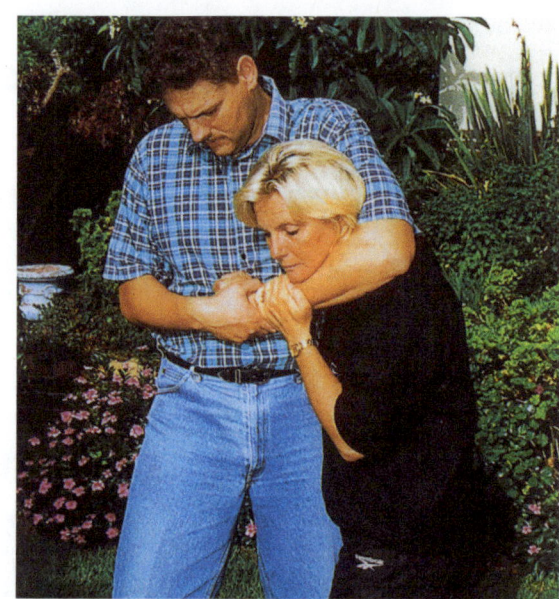

2. Fling your arm behind, up and over the attacker's shoulder that is closest to you. Hook your thumb (or fingers) underneath his jaw and push his head backwards.

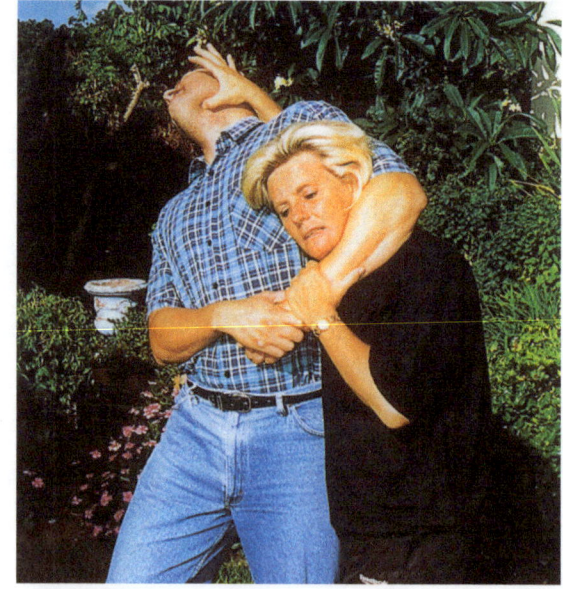

SELF-DEFENCE SCENARIOS

3 Keep pushing until he loosens his grip, then push his arm away from your neck.

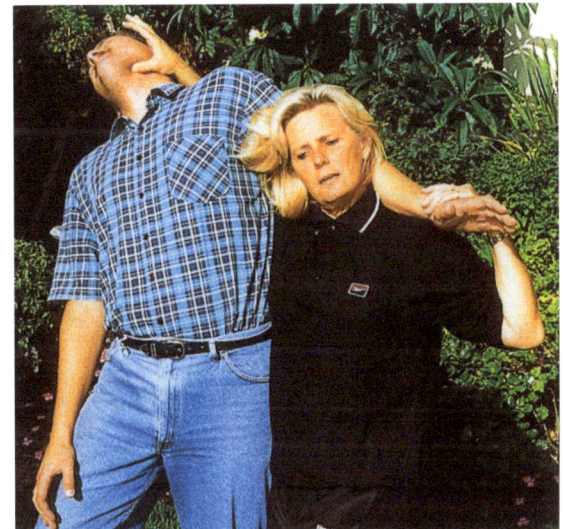

4 With the palm of your hand, strike down hard into his groin.

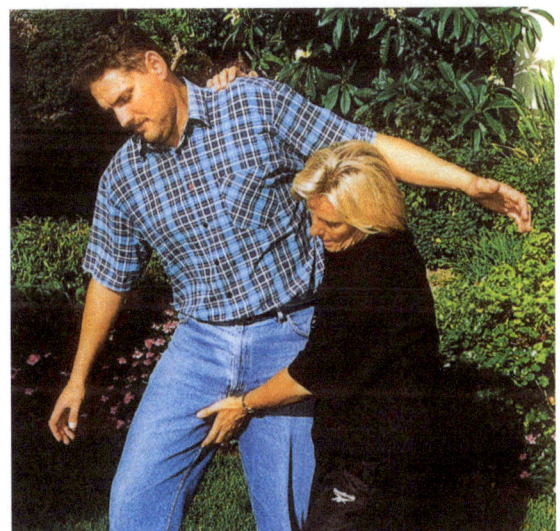

◀ **TIPS**

» Don't panic. Initially it may feel as if there is nothing you can do. However, the thumb-under-jaw technique is very effective.

STRANGLEHOLD WITH ONE ARM AROUND THE NECK (2)

1 Your assailant grabs you around the neck with one arm and locks his hands.

2 Fling your arm behind, up and over the attacker's shoulder that is closest to you. Place your strongest finger between his upper lip and nose.

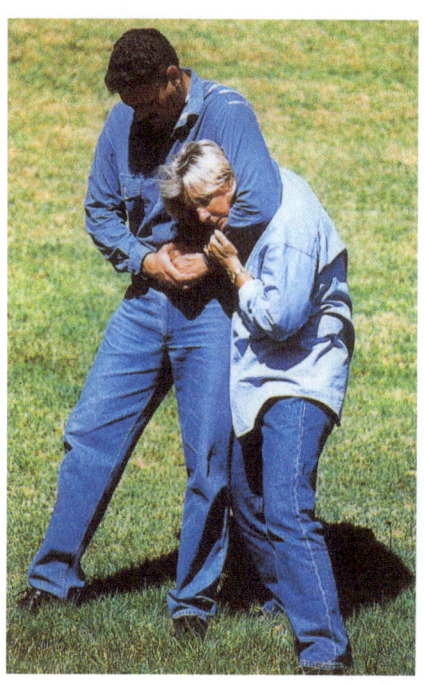

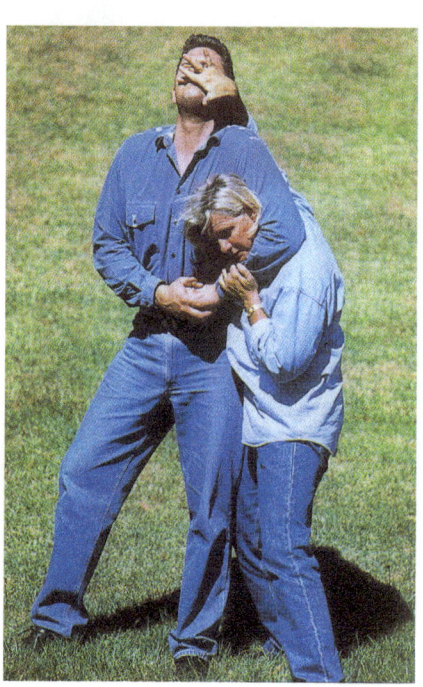

3 Push your hand backwards until he releases his grip on you.

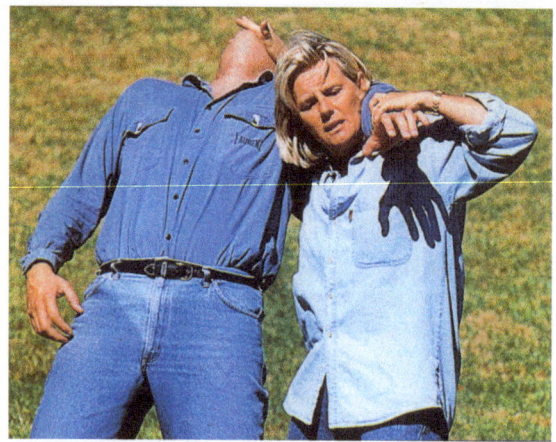

SELF-DEFENCE SCENARIOS

4 Completely remove yourself from his grip.

5 Strike with the palm of your hand down onto his groin.

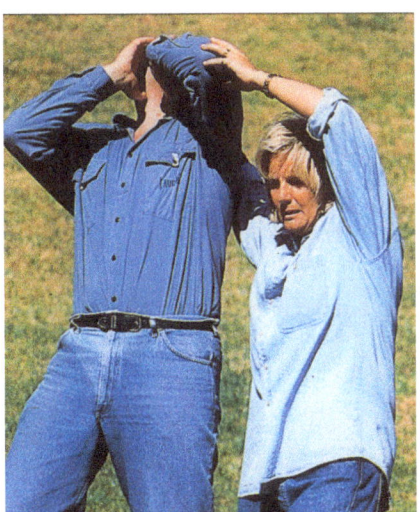

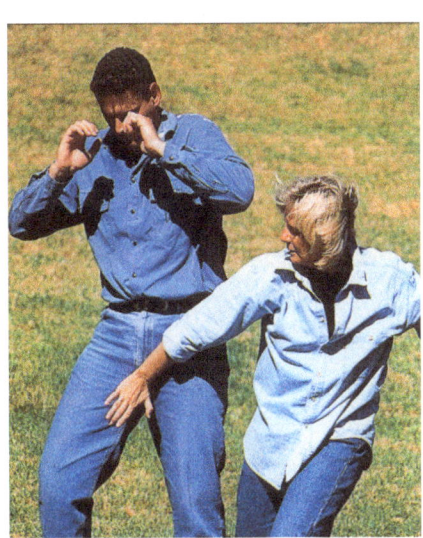

6 Wind up with your elbow and strike down hard onto the back of his neck.

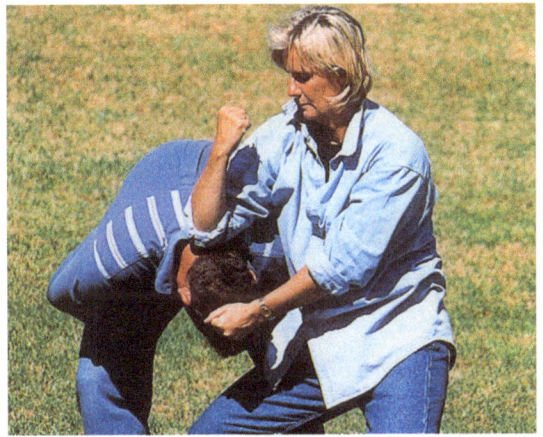

◀ TIPS

» Although you can't see what you're doing because of the way you are being held, your attacker's nose is an easy target to feel for. Once you have located it, place a finger directly under it and push hard (see Basic Self-Defence Techniques, page 80).

STRANGLEHOLD WITH ONE ARM AROUND THE NECK (3)

1 Your assailant approaches you from the side.

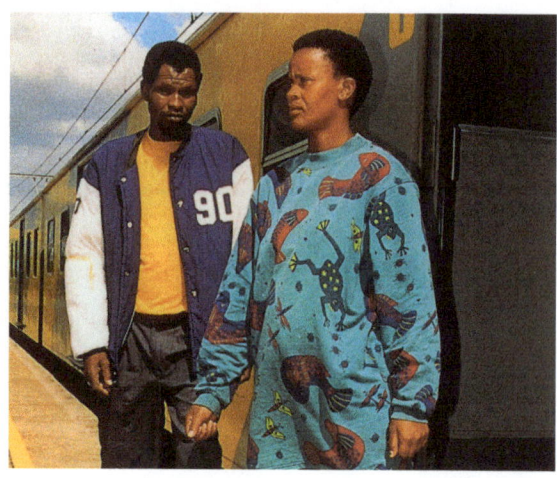

2 He grabs hold of your neck with one arm. Wind up by bringing your hand towards your shoulder.

3 Strike down hard with your arm or the side of your hand between your assailant's legs.

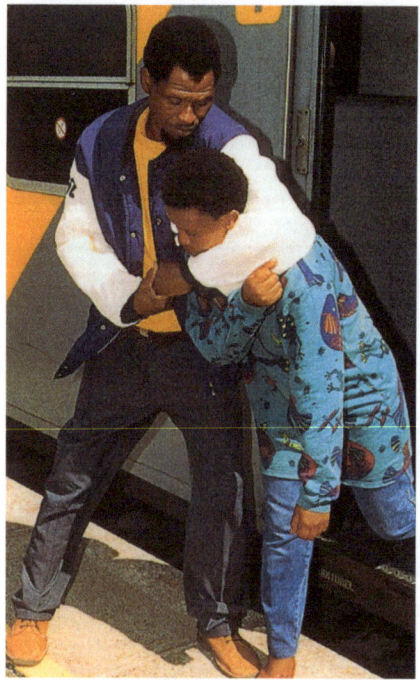

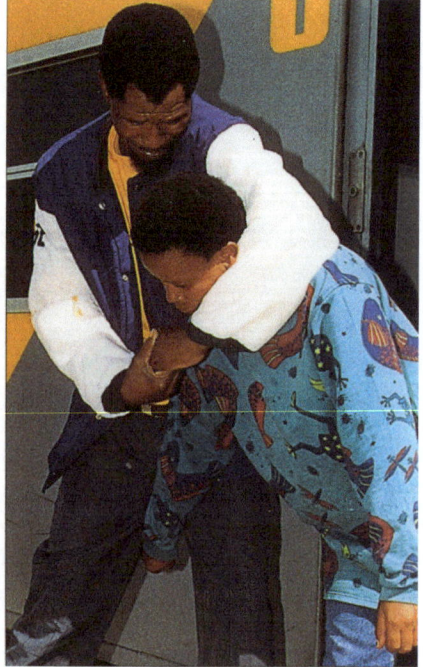

SELF-DEFENCE SCENARIOS

4 Pull your hand back again, up towards your shoulder, as a wind up for your follow-up technique.

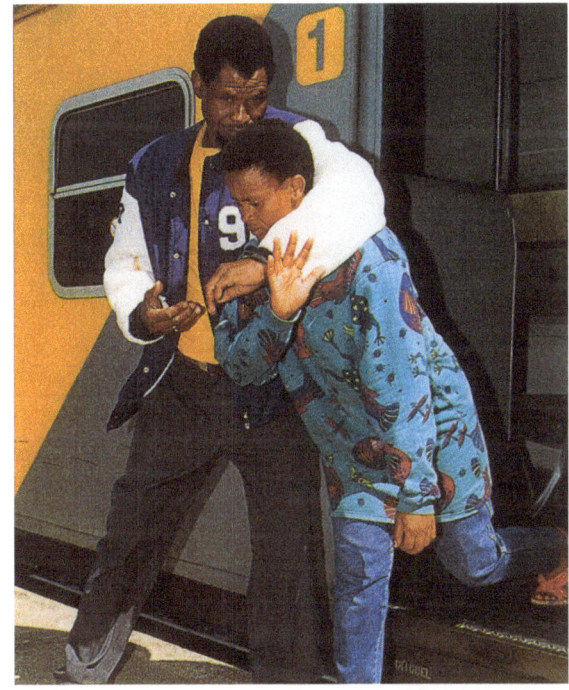

5 Your assailant will have released his grip by the time your hand is moving downward for your next technique. Hit your assailant between his legs with your arm, then grab his groin and pull hard.

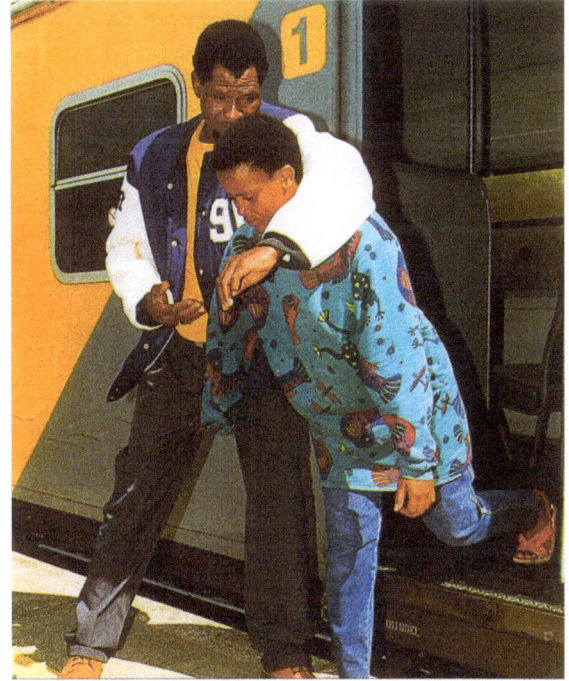

ATTACK TO THE THROAT WITH BOTH HANDS

In certain situations, you may be positioned quite a bit lower than your assailant at the time of the attack. This is usually the case when you are attacked while sitting down. Because of this awkward position, his arms will quite often obstruct a clear strike to his face. Striking him in his groin first will bring him down, thereby making his face more accessible for follow-up techniques.

1. Your assailant attacks you from the side by grabbing your throat.

2. His arms are in the way and prevent a clear strike to his face, therefore, strike downward with your hand onto his groin.

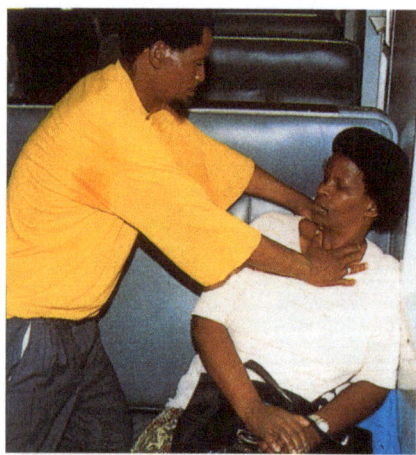
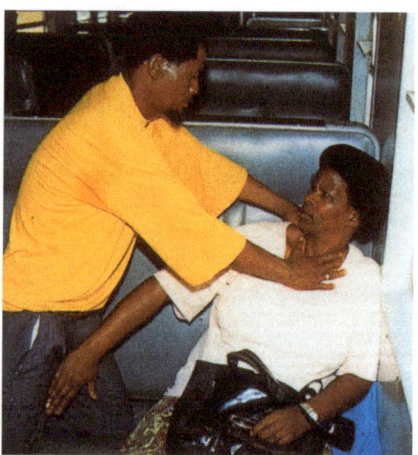

3. As your assailant drops his hands, snap your arm back towards your body as a wind up, and make a fist.

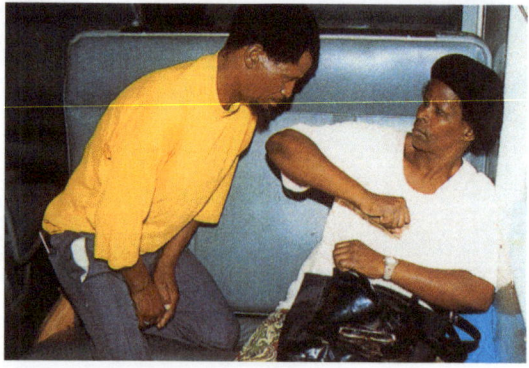

SELF-DEFENCE SCENARIOS

4 Hit your assailant's hard nose with the knuckles of your fist.

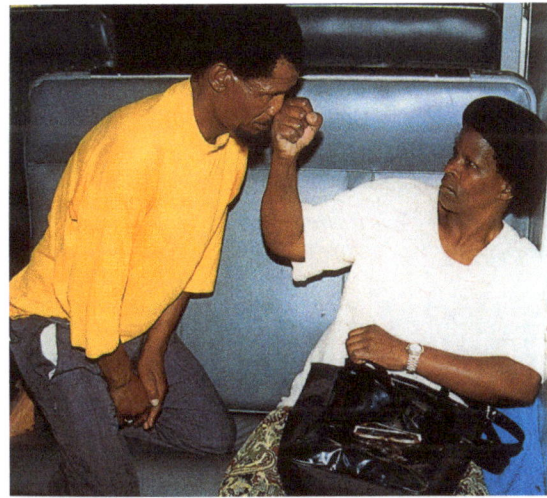

5 Get up quickly from your seat and push your assailant away.

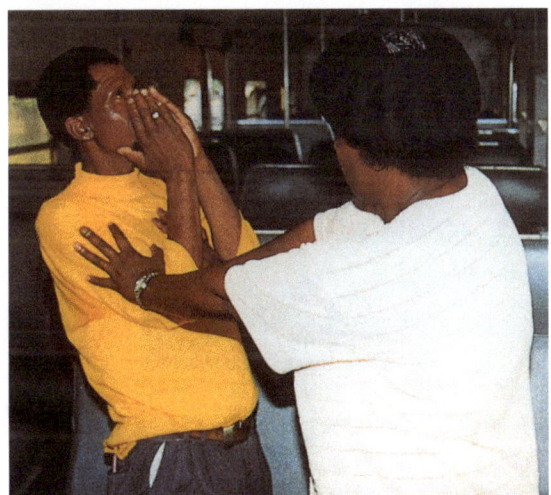

◀ TIPS

» If you are struggling to breathe, DON'T PANIC. Implement your self-defence techniques as quickly as possible to force him to release his grip around your neck.
» The downward strike to his groin can be made with either the outer edge of your hand or with a closed fist.

ATTACK WHILE SITTING DOWN

1 The assailant places his hand on your leg. Wind up with your elbow.

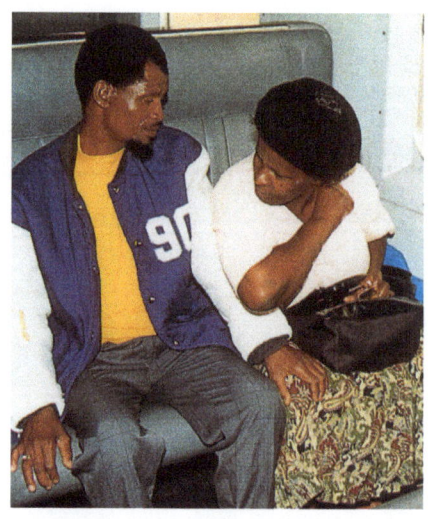

OPTION A: Bring your elbow back in a hard strike on his throat.

OPTION B: Bring your elbow back hard onto his nose.

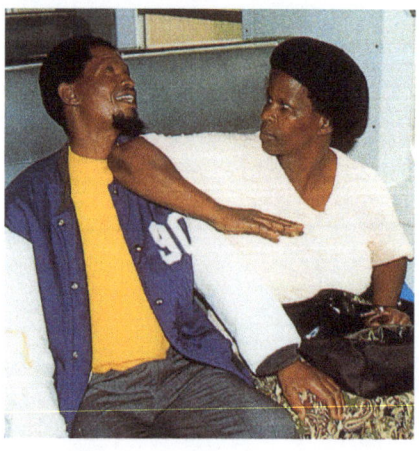
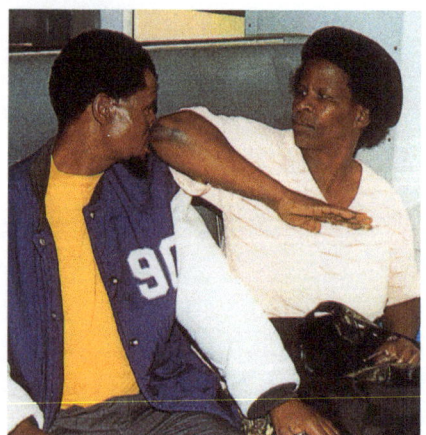

> ◀ **TIPS**
>
> » The elbow is a wonderfully effective self-defence tool. It is the ideal close-range weapon (inside a car, lift, etc.)

SELF-DEFENCE SCENARIOS

ATTACKS ON THE GROUND AND LYING DOWN

ATTACK TO THE BODY WITH BOTH HANDS

This type of approach would be very typical of a fantasy rapist. If it is a fantasy rapist, it is also possible that he will be naked. Don't panic. Take advantage of the fact that all his target areas are completely exposed and unprotected.

1 Your assailant grabs your shoulder and your leg.

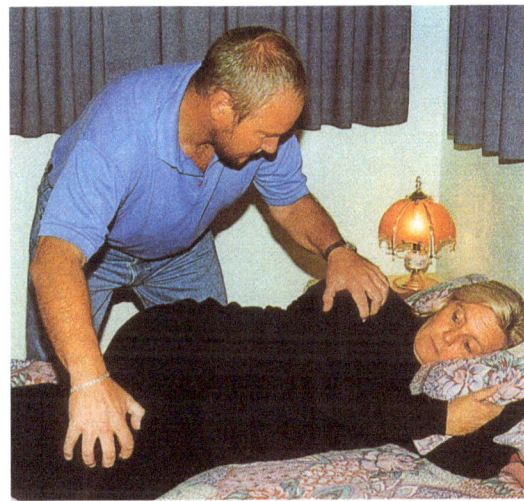

2 He turns your body towards him.

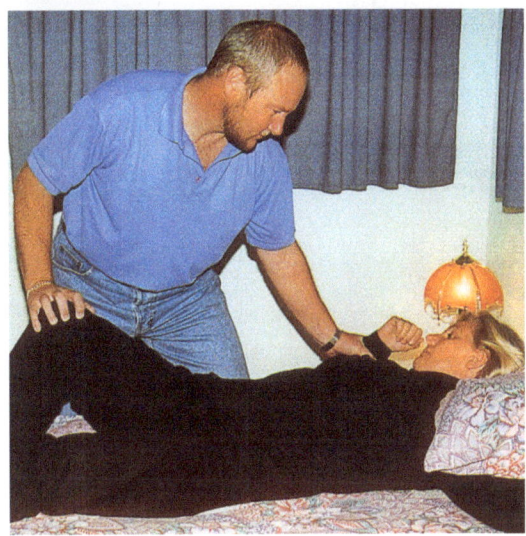

THE SOUTH AFRICAN WOMEN'S GUIDE TO SELF-DEFENCE

3 He pins your wrist down and tries to swing his leg over your body.

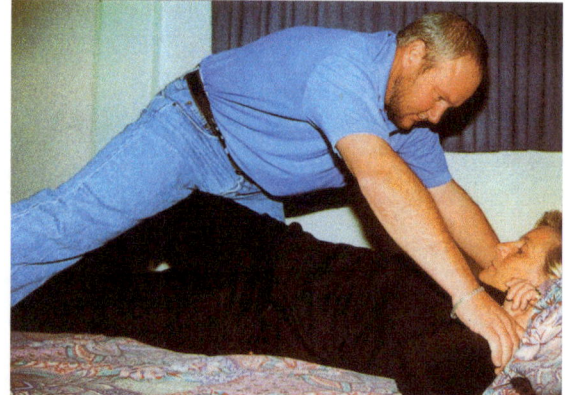

4 As he moves his leg across your body, lift your knee up.

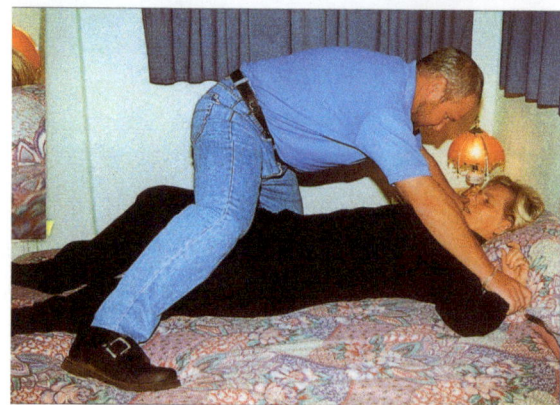

5 Jab your assailant with your knee between his legs and into his groin.

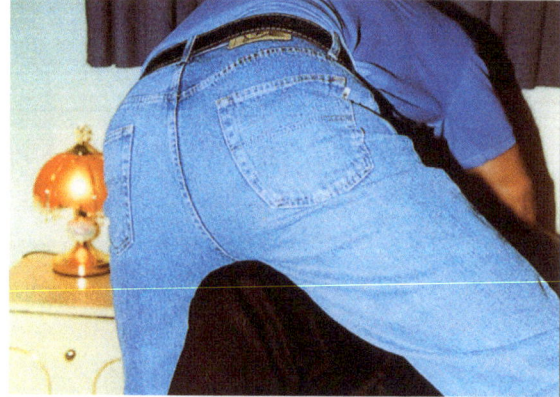

SELF-DEFENCE SCENARIOS

6 Lift up your leg as the wind up for your next technique.

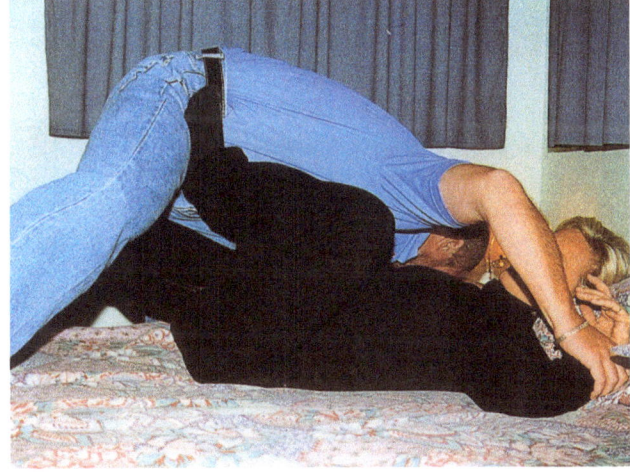

7 Kick your assailant away from you.

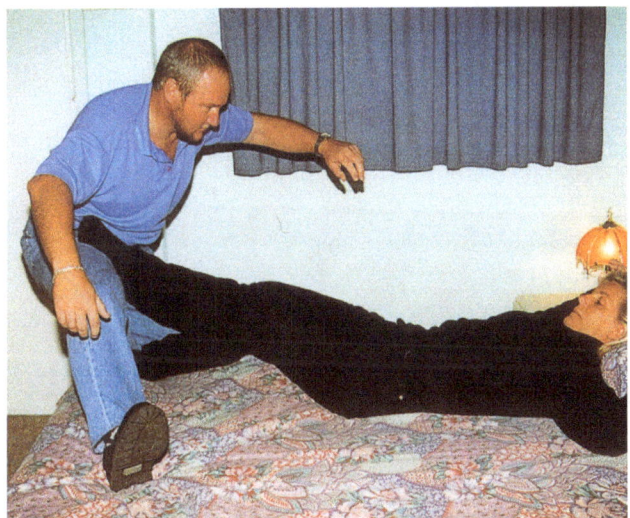

◀ TIPS

» Your first priority is to get your attacker off you and to get up into a standing position. Once off, you can follow up with other basic self-defence techniques.

ATTACK TO THE THROAT WITH BOTH HANDS (1)

1. Your assailant strangles you with both hands.

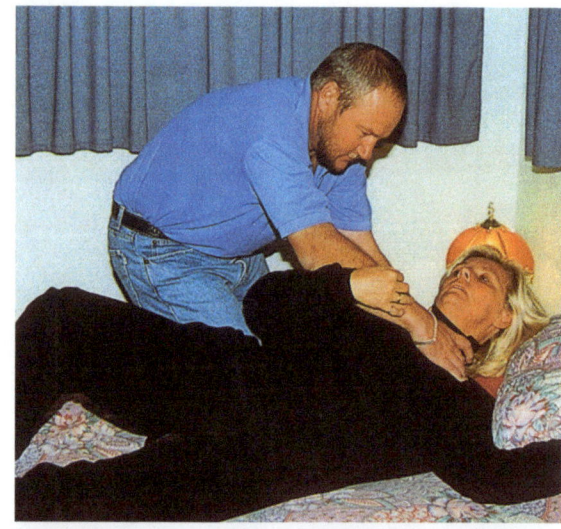

2. Poke your strongest finger into his throat (just below his Adam's apple).

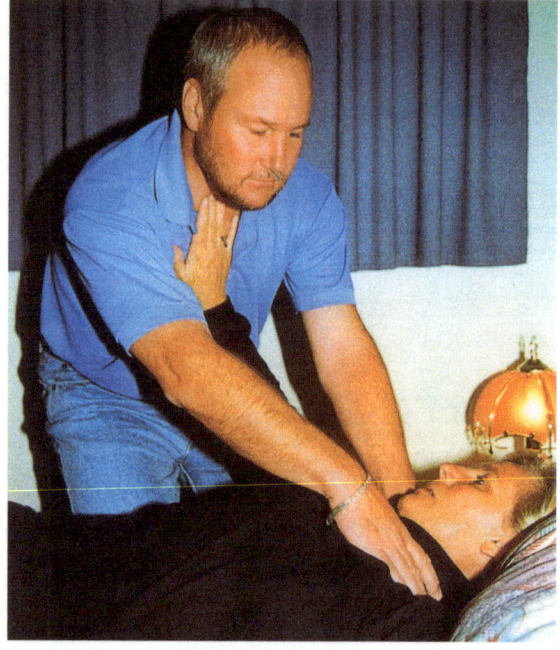

SELF-DEFENCE SCENARIOS

3 Keeping your finger there, push hard against this sensitive area of his throat.

4 Wind up with your elbow.

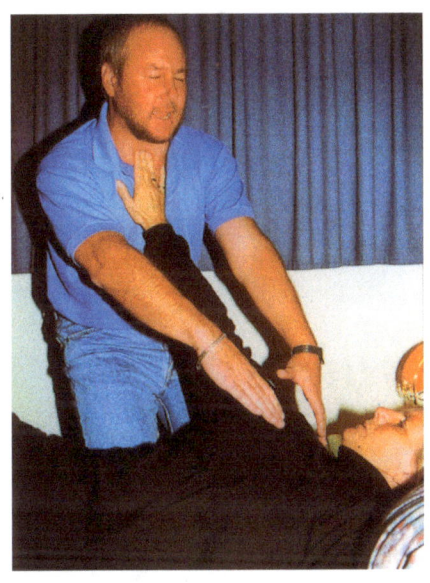

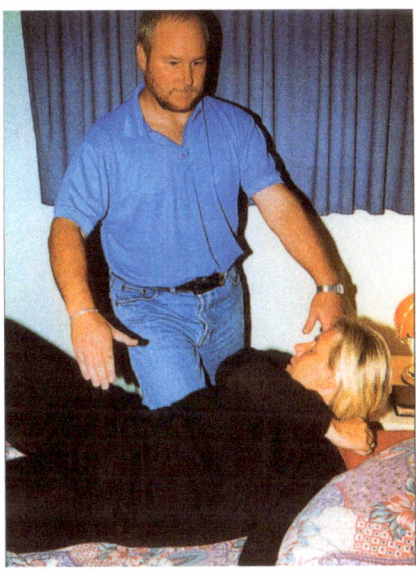

5 Strike your assailant's groin hard with your elbow.

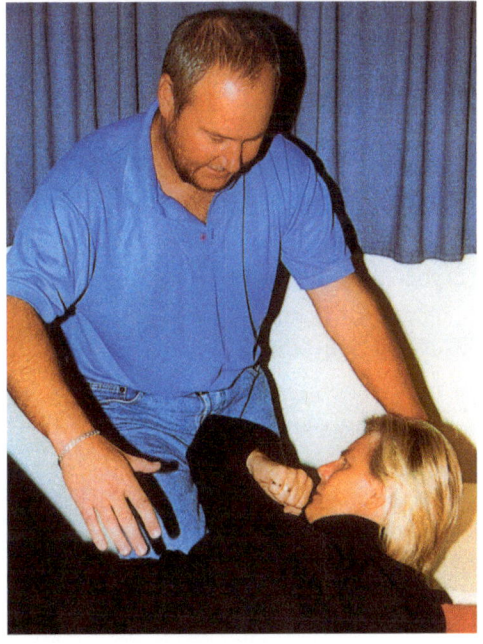

ATTACK TO THE THROAT WITH BOTH HANDS (2)

1. Your assailant is strangling you with both hands.

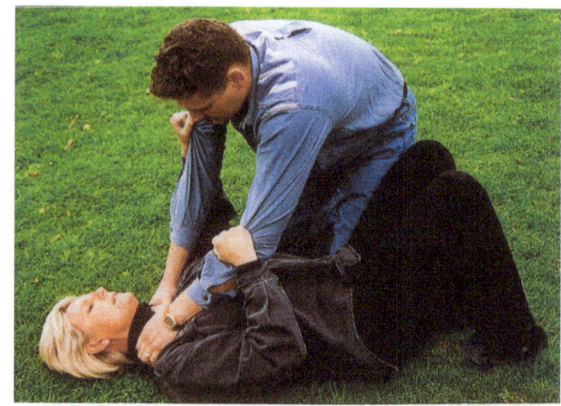

2. Swing your leg up and hook it around your assailant's neck.

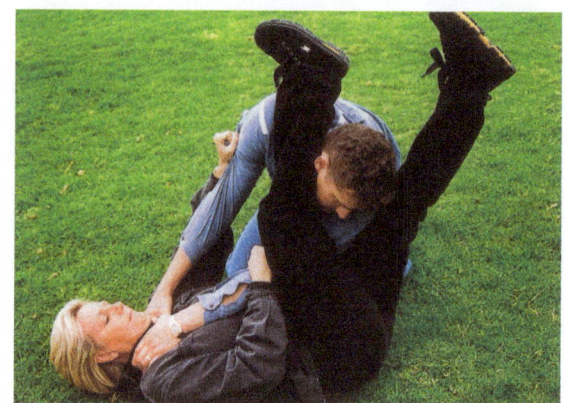

3. Using your leg, pull your assailant's head down to the ground. Pull yourself into a sitting position by gripping hold of his arms.

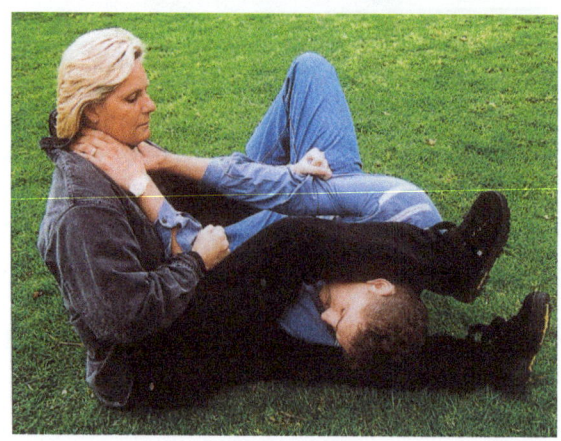

SELF-DEFENCE SCENARIOS

OPTION A:

4 Swing your leg up for momentum and impact while still holding onto your assailant.

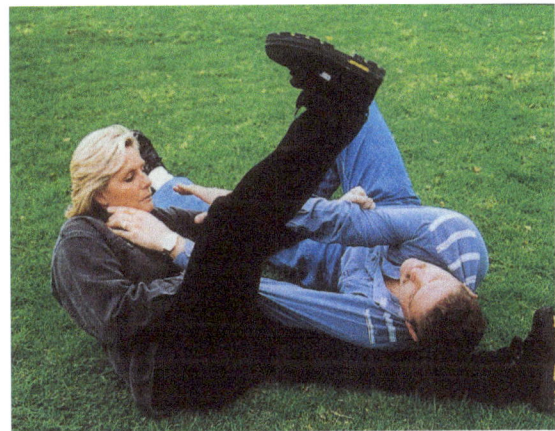

5 Kick your heel down hard onto your assailant's nose.

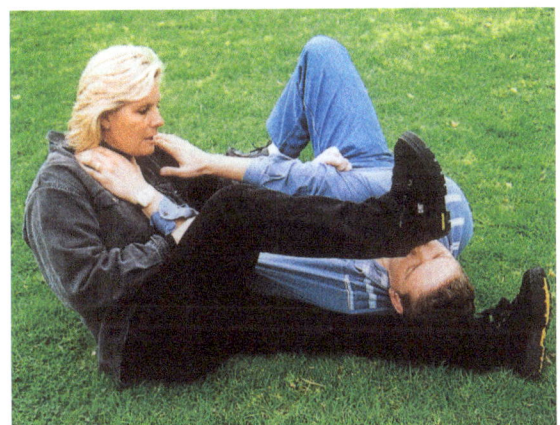

◀ TIPS

» In step 2, the left leg can stay on the ground. In other words, both legs do not have to be lifted.
» Get up off the ground as quickly as possible and get away.
» If your hands cannot reach your attacker, use your legs. This is illustrated in the downward kick to the face (Option A, step 5).

OPTION B:

4 Once in a sitting position, hold onto your assailant's arm and bend it backwards.

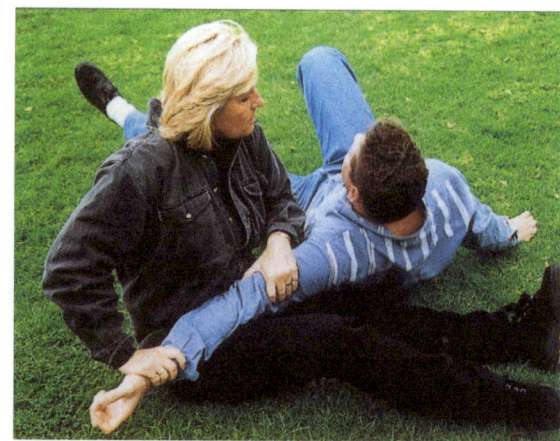

5 Still holding his arm, wind up high with your other elbow.

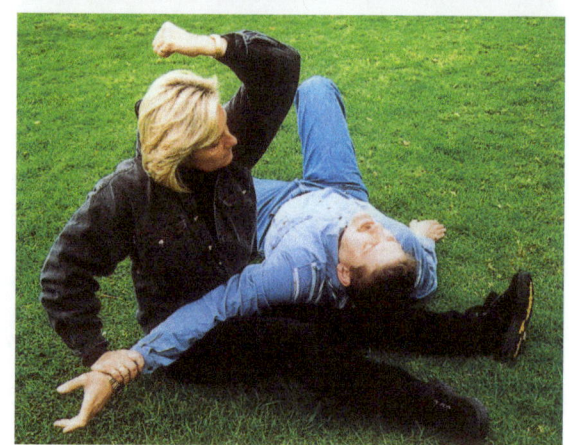

6 Using this elbow, strike down hard onto his nose.

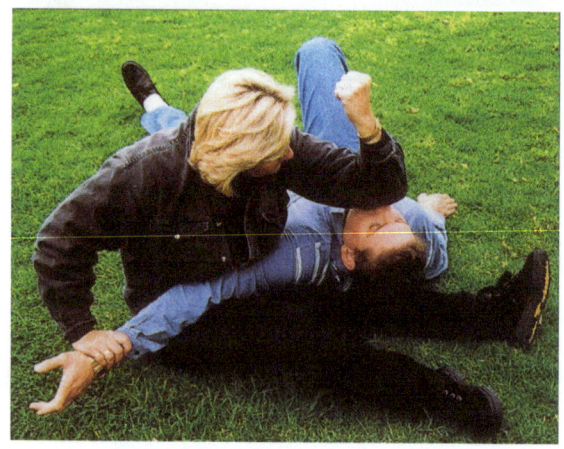

SELF-DEFENCE SCENARIOS

ATTACK TO THE THROAT WITH BOTH HANDS (3)

1. Your assailant has thrown you down onto the ground and is strangling you with both hands.

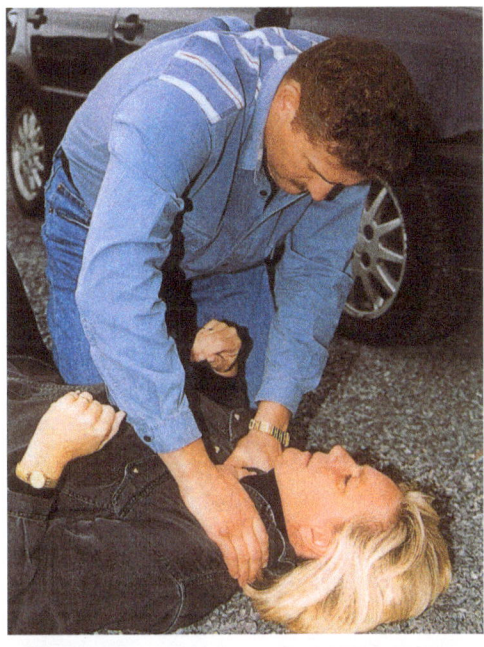

OPTION A:

2. **If he is on your right side:**
Slide your right arm up underneath his arm towards his neck and grab hold of his shirt collar. Bring your left arm up on the outside, crossing it over your right arm, and grab the collar on the other side of his neck. (There will be a cross-action with your arms.)

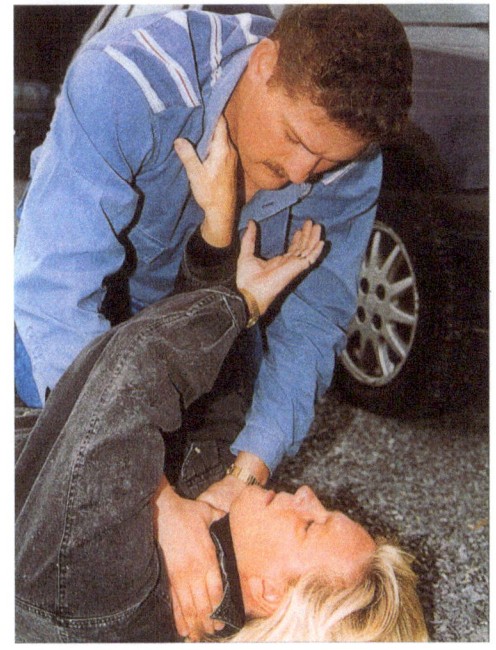

155

3 With both of your hands still crossed, tighten your hold on his shirt in a stranglehold grip. This can be done by pulling your hands together.

4 Using your grip on his shirt to support your next movement, slide the lower part of your body out and away from your assailant in an anti-clockwise direction by pedaling your feet on the ground. Keep doing this until your face is no longer underneath his body. Keep your hands in the cross-locked position all the time.

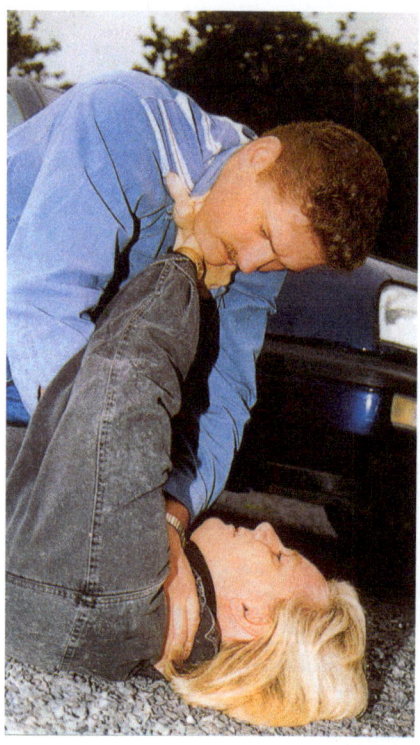

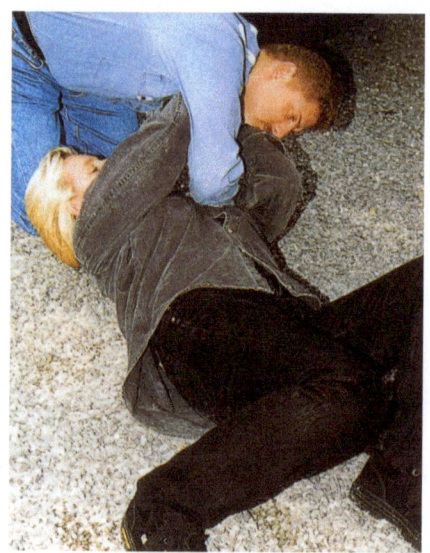

5 Your assailant will fall over.

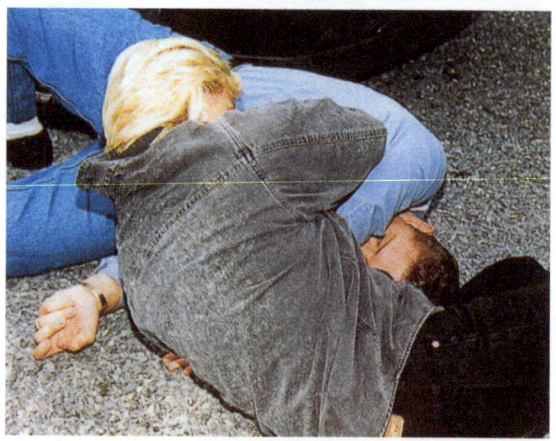

SELF-DEFENCE SCENARIOS

6 Swing your body up into a sitting position while still holding onto his shirt.

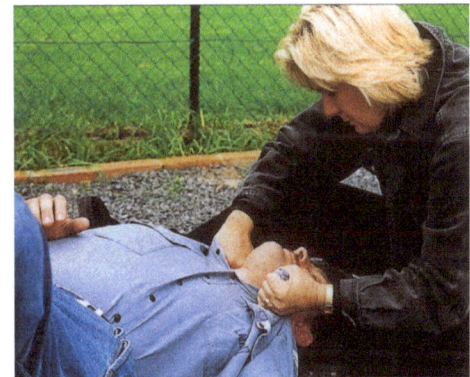

7 Wind up high with your elbow.

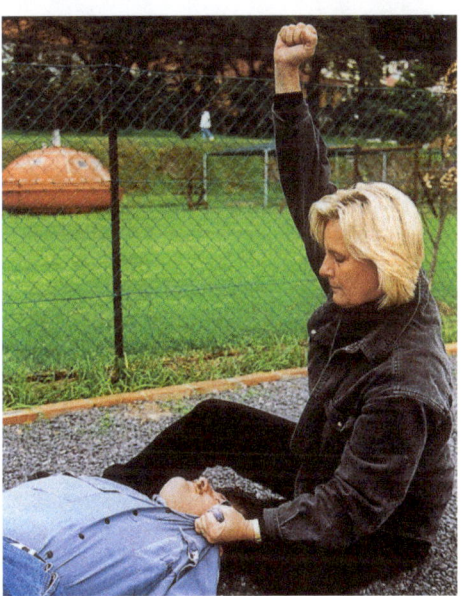

8 Using this elbow, hit down hard onto your assailant's nose.

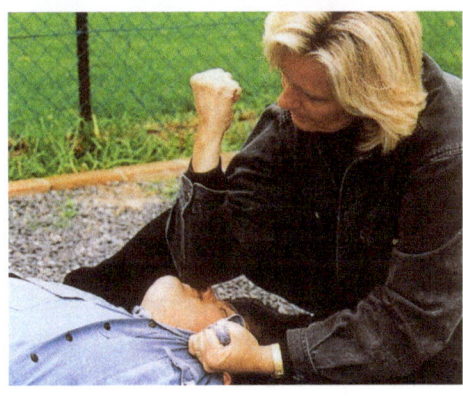

OPTION B:

2 Punch the assailant's nose hard.

3 Continue to use suitable follow-up techniques, such as hitting hard onto his ears, poking your fingers into his eyes or punching into his groin.

OPTION C:

2 Poke your strong fingers into your assailant's throat (just below his Adam's apple). Dig in your fingers and push back hard until he releases his grip.

3 Continue to use suitable follow-up techniques, such as punching into his groin.

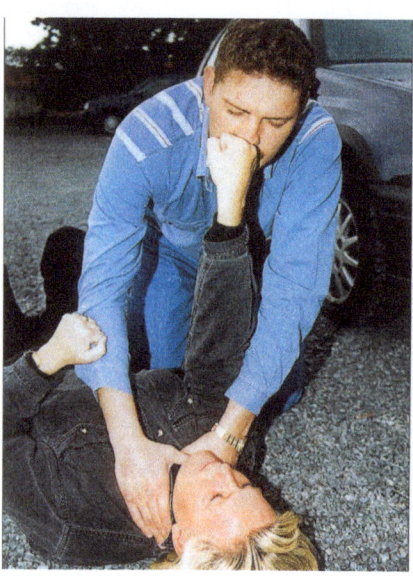
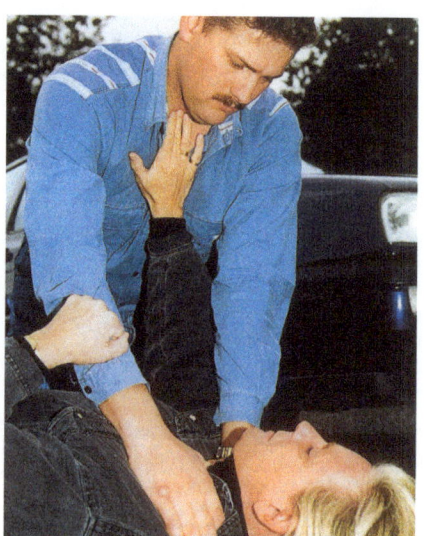

OPTION D:

2 Strike the assailant's groin using the palm of your hand. You can then also grab and pull.

3 Continue to use suitable follow-up techniques, such as hitting hard onto his ears or poking your fingers into his eyes.

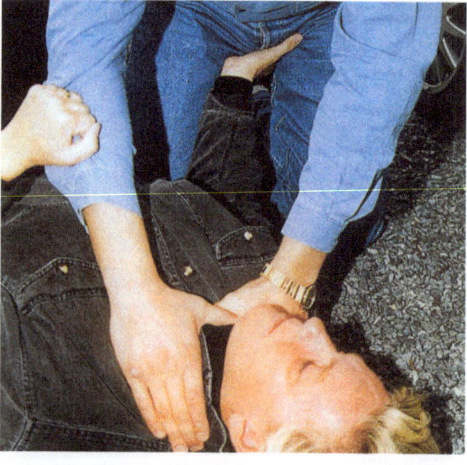

SELF-DEFENCE SCENARIOS

GENERAL GROUND TECHNIQUE (1)

This technique (known as the pedaling technique) is very effective if you missed your opportunity to implement a knee-to-groin technique when your assailant first placed his leg between yours. In some instances, the angle and position of the attacker's body also makes it too awkward to implement a knee-to-groin technique, especially if his body is too close to yours.

The purpose of this technique is to prevent him placing both of his legs between yours. This is not only precisely where he wants to be, but it will make a knee-to-groin technique extremely difficult, if not impossible.

At some stage during the pedaling technique, your attacker will have to lift his body enough to allow you to finally implement your knee-to-groin technique. Because he will always have one knee on the ground while the other is up in the air, you may have an opportunity to unbalance him and force him to fall over on one side.

◀ TIPS

» If you have weak knees or any kind of knee injury, it is recommended that another ground technique is used instead of this one, as it could lead to further damage.

1. Your assailant has thrown you to the ground.

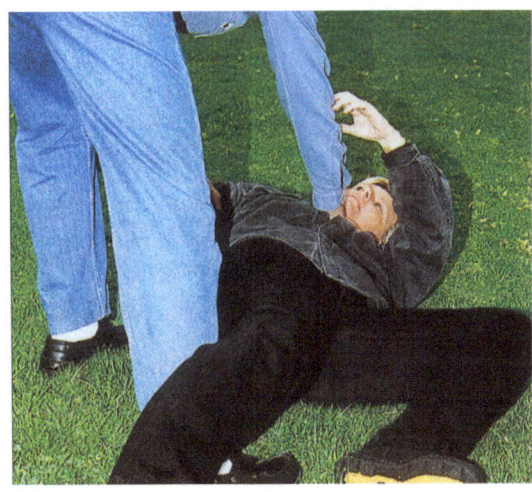

THE SOUTH AFRICAN WOMEN'S GUIDE TO SELF-DEFENCE

2 He pins your wrists down and puts one leg (first leg) down between your legs. Curl your leg around the leg he has just placed between your legs and hook your foot underneath it.

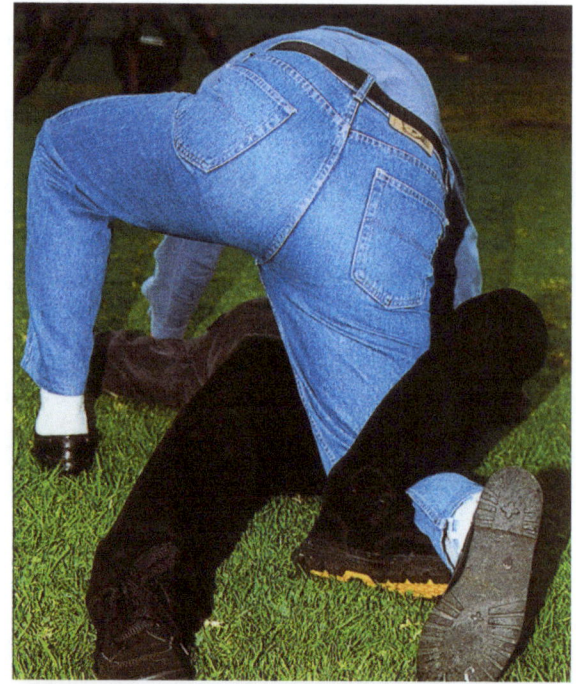

3 As he tries to get his other leg (second leg) between yours, lift up your other leg to prevent his leg from securing its position.

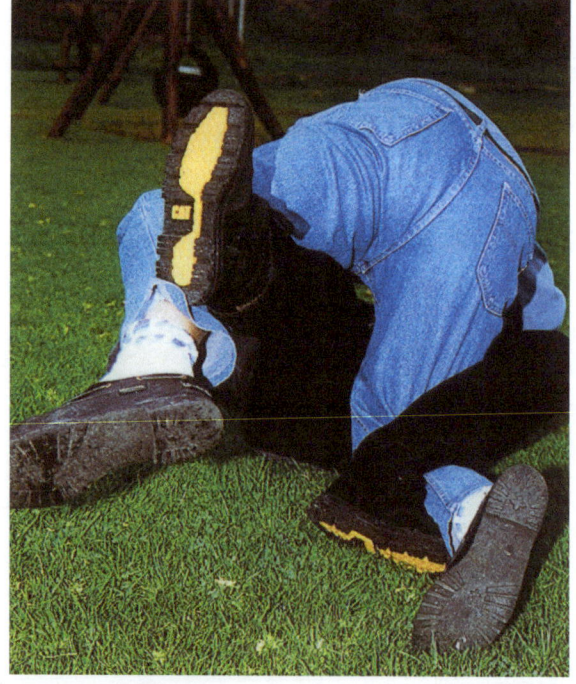

SELF-DEFENCE SCENARIOS

4 If he lifts his leg higher, lift yours too. Keep your other leg hooked around his first leg all the time.

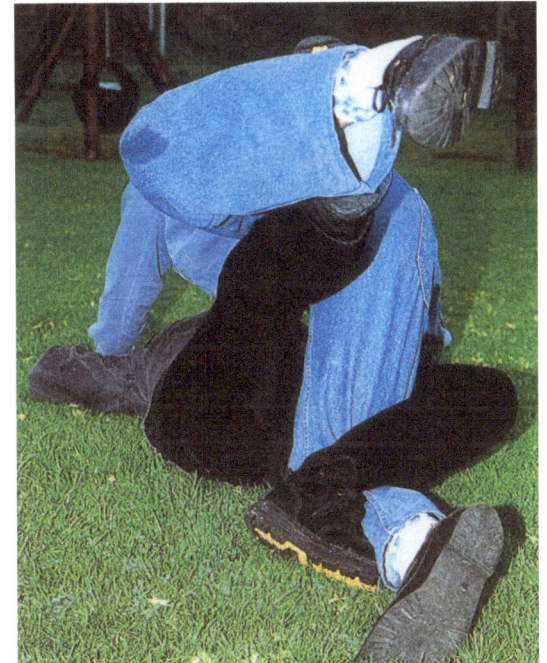

5 As he struggles to get his second leg over your free leg, he will put this leg onto the ground, and try to lift his first leg. You must lift the foot that is locked around this leg, too, so that he is unable to do anything with his leg.

6 He will swop back to his second leg in yet another effort to get it over yours and between your legs. Again, you must lift your second leg with his. This creates a 'pedalling' motion. It is helpful to work within the rhythm of his movements. As he lifts, so you lift. As he drops, so you drop.

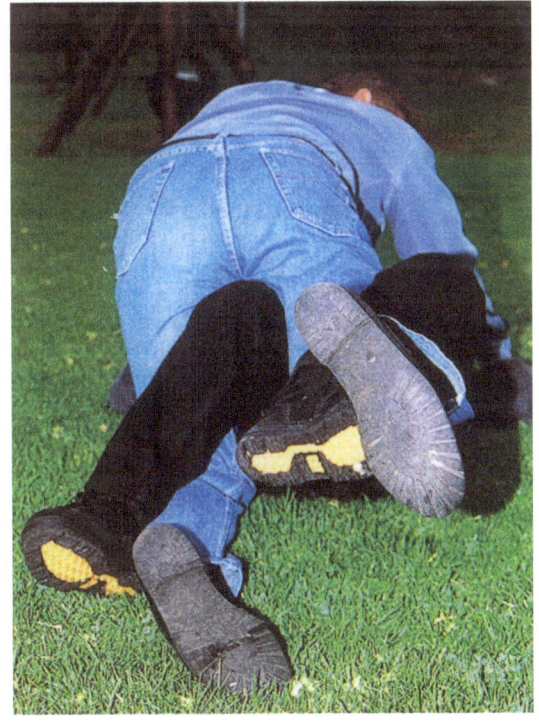

THE SOUTH AFRICAN WOMEN'S GUIDE TO SELF-DEFENCE

GENERAL GROUND TECHNIQUE (2)

1. As your assailant passes you, he grabs you around the throat with one arm and throws you down.

2. The moment you hit the ground, grab a handful of sand and throw it into your assailant's eyes.

3. While he is temporarily immobilized, get up quickly and run away.

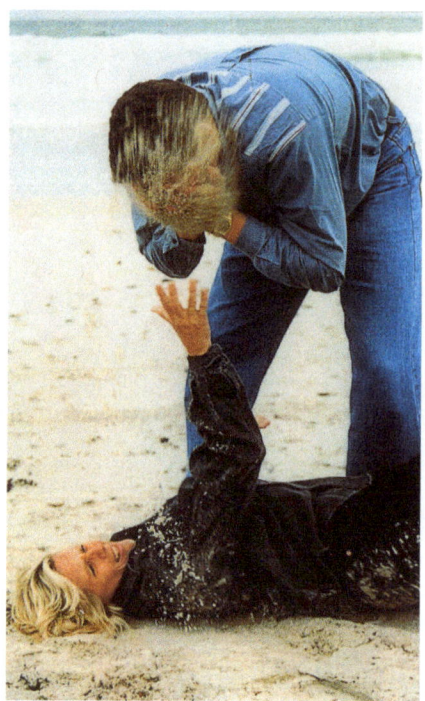

◀ TIPS

» If you feel that you cannot get up quickly enough to run away, pull your knee back and kick him in his groin. If he topples forward, be careful he does not fall on top of you. OR, pull both your legs back and kick towards him in an effort to push him backwards onto his back. You will now have time to get up and run away.

GENERAL GROUND TECHNIQUE (3)

1. Your attacker has pushed you to the ground. He is standing at your feet with one foot on either side of yours. Hook your feet around his leg.

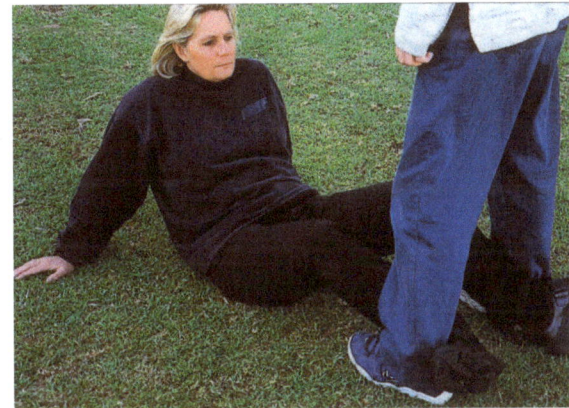

2. With a fast, strong action, move your feet apart and pull them towards you.

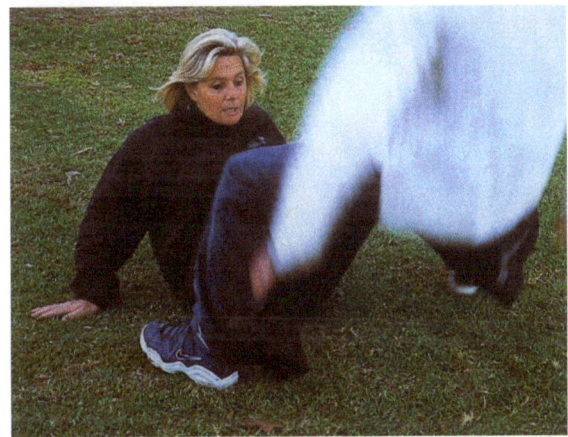

3. Your attacker will fall onto his back. Lift your one leg as a wind up for your next technique.

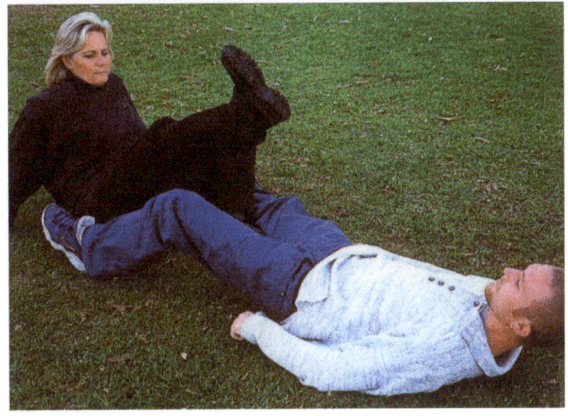

4 Bring your foot down hard onto his groin.

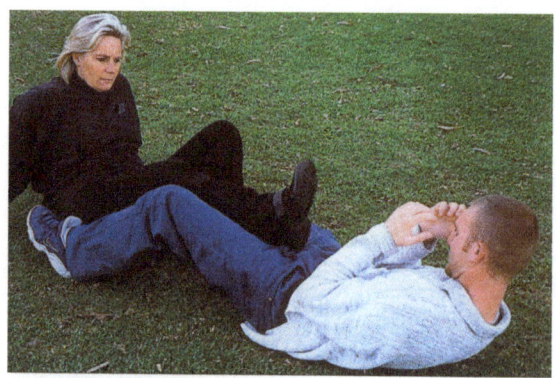

GETTING UP OFF THE GROUND

1 If you fall to the ground, lock your legs together and keep them locked if at all possible.

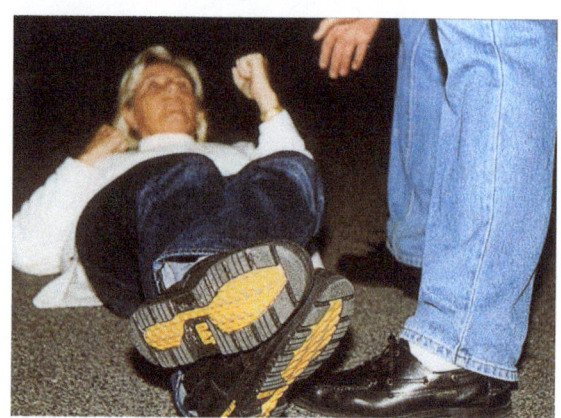

2 Keep your hands free for defence.

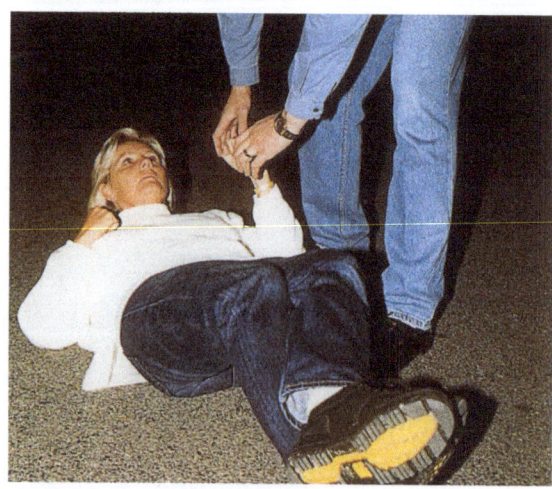

SELF-DEFENCE SCENARIOS

3 Bring your upper body into an upright position without allowing your hands to touch the ground. This is to keep your hands free for defence and attack techniques.

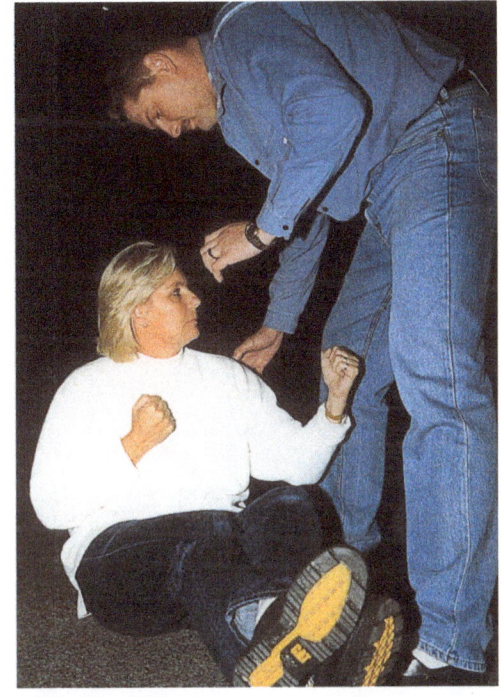

OPTION A:

4 As your assailant moves within striking distance, punch hard into his groin.

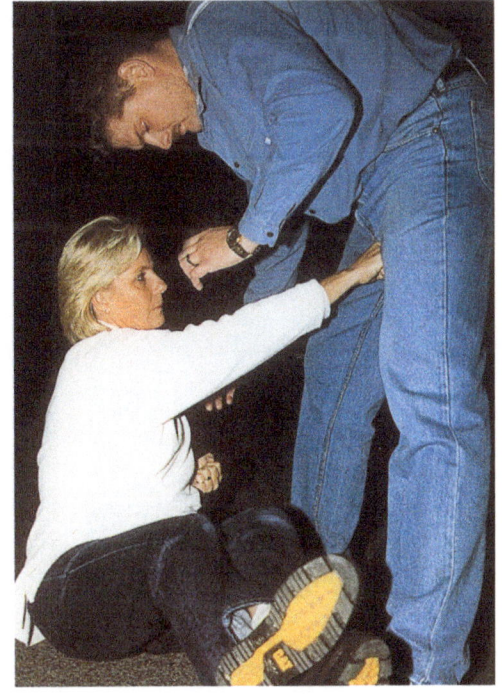

5 The assailant will react to the blow, which will give you a chance to quickly shift your body from a sitting position into a position on your feet.

6 Punch your assailant in the groin again.

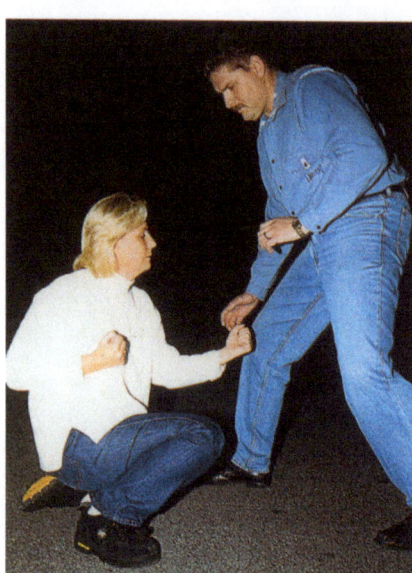
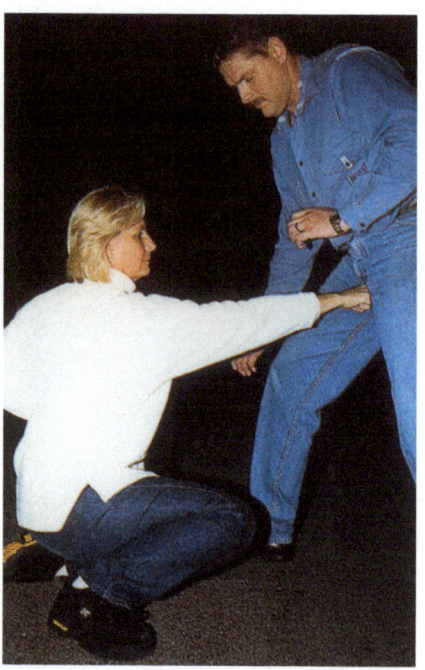

7 Shift your body from its low position into an upright stance and punch your assailant hard on his nose.

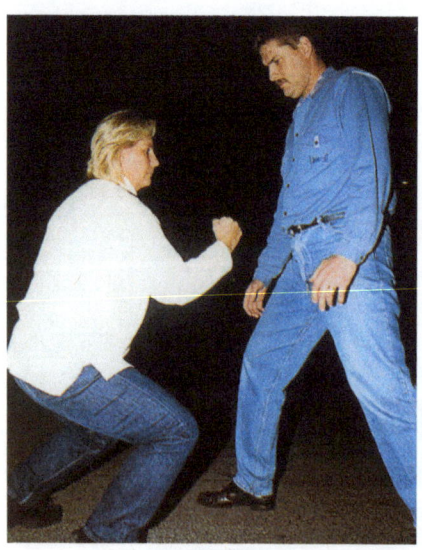
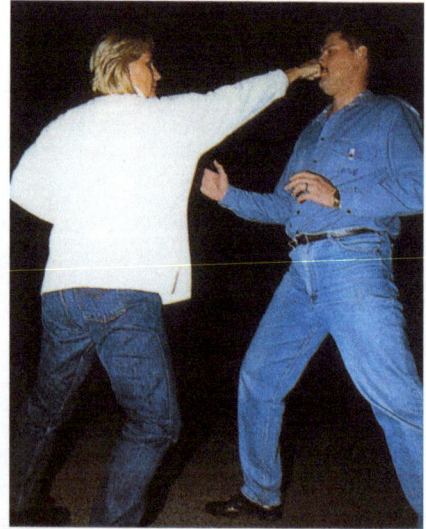

SELF-DEFENCE SCENARIOS

OPTION B:

4 With legs still locked, use your arms for defence.

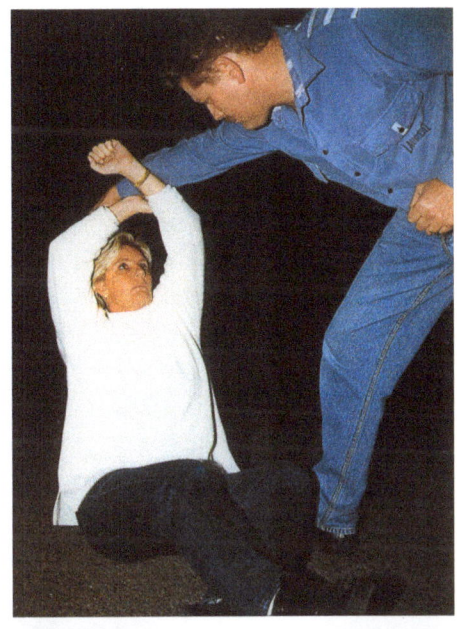

5 Your arms can support your body for balance as you kick up into your assailant's groin.

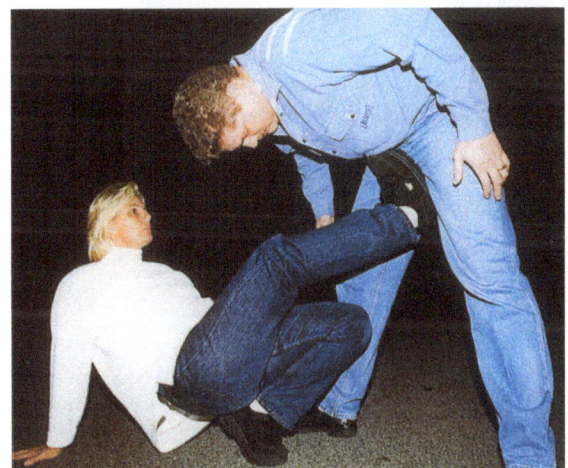

◀ TIPS

- » Always try to get up off the ground as quickly as possible.
- » Keep your hands free at all times for defence.
- » Keep your eyes focused on your attacker at all times.

7
OBJECTS AS WEAPONS

When you make the decision to fight back to prevent being raped, you must be prepared to do whatever it takes and to use whatever you can to assist you. There is nothing wrong with using weapons if you feel that they will increase your chances of survival.

All homes and offices have objects that can be used as weapons. These can be thrown, smashed over your attacker's head or sprayed into his face.

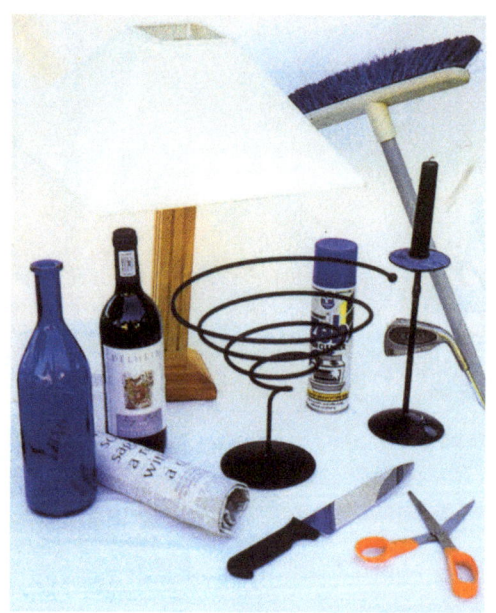

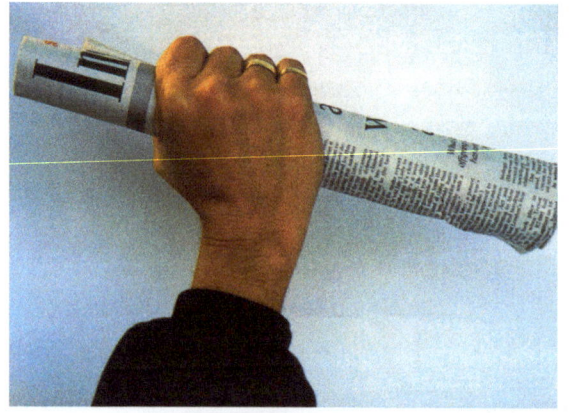

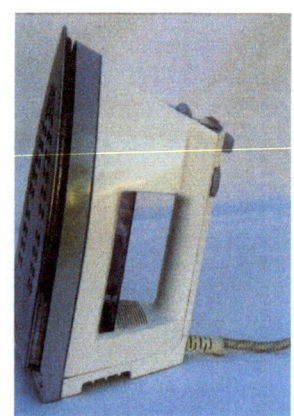

OBJECTS AS WEAPONS

Even the average handbag has suitable weapons in it, such as a pen or a set of car keys.

If you're at home and you hear a noise (someone trying to enter your home or circling the perimeter), immediately pick up something you can use as a weapon and call the nearest reaction unit or the police. Your weapon could be a knife, a letter opener, a vase or heavy ceramic pot, a golf club, a metal candlestick holder, an aerosol can, mace spray, or anything else around you that is suitable. Look at ALL your options.

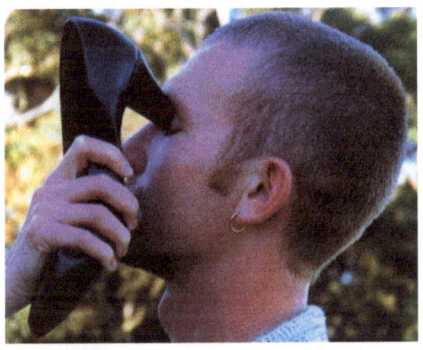

A high-heeled shoe can be used as a very effective weapon.

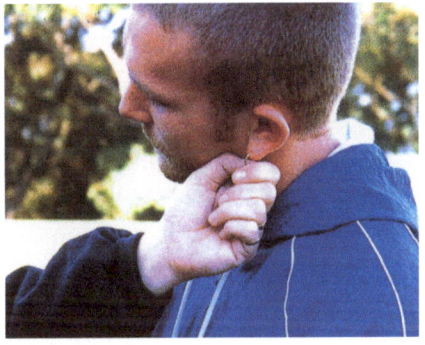

If your attacker is wearing an earring, grab it and pull hard.

Other useful weapons are:
» a rolled-up newspaper (to jab)
» a broom (to jab and/or hit)
» an ashtray (to throw)
» a kitchen knife
» pepper (to throw in his eyes)
» a pair of scissors
» a bottle
» high-heeled shoes (strike into his face with the heel)
» your attacker's own earring, if he's wearing any (pull)
» a set of car keys (splayed and gripped between your fingers and used to slash across his face or poke into his eyes).

ACKNOWLEDGMENTS

Vanessa Wilson, Pieter Smit (photographer), Margaret Neethling, Herman Bosman, Shane Lucas, Veronica Mann, Karen Johnson, Chrislene Smith, Darlene Lubbe, Florence Harding, Fritz Carelse, Marguerite Esterhuizen, Glynis Marais, Denis Skeate, Constance Gxowa, Eliza Gwabile, John Nogilana, Carol Bower (Director, RAPCAN, Cape Town), Chantel Cooper (Director, Rape Crisis Cape Town), Dr L J Martin (Chief Specialist/Head of Division, Forensic Medicine & Toxicology, University of Cape Town), Marcel Londt (Child Abuse Therapeutic & Training Services cc), Elsabe Durr Fitschen (Clinical Social Worker), Lilly Artz (Gender, Health and Justice Research Unit, University of Cape Town), Vanessa Raphaely (Editor, *Cosmopolitan* magazine) for launching the Cosmo Kicks Butt self-defence workshops in 2001 with her wonderful team of Cosmo-girls and driving the programme with such passion and fervor, Kathy Rath (Rape Survivor, Port Elizabeth) for sharing her experience with us, Brian Weyers (Marketing Director, Shoprite Checkers) and Maryke Visser (Public Relations & GSI Manager, Shoprite Group of Companies) for their support of, and commitment to, the Shoprite Self-defence Training Programme for female learners in the Western Cape since the launch of the programme in 2003.

SPECIAL THANKS

A sincere thank you to all the rape survivors, past and present, that have so honestly and generously shared their stories with me, providing the information that has formed a large part of the research for this book – in particular, Lois Wagner.

To Pieter Smit, who did an outstanding job with the photography and who patiently shot what seemed like an endless stream of scenarios and techniques.

ACKNOWLEDGMENTS

To all my friends for their love and continued support over the years – it is much appreciated.

Finally, I would like to offer a special thank you to my right hand PeeWee (Vanessa Wilson), for her hours of hard work on this book and her unselfish contribution to, and belief in, my work from the beginning. Not only does she appreciate and understand the passion that I have for what I am doing, but she also has a wonderful talent for understanding and putting down, so accurately in words, what it is that I want to say and how I'd like to say it. I really couldn't have wished for anyone better to have worked with on this book.

RESOURCES

SELF-DEFENCE & RAPE PREVENTION WORKSHOPS

Stay Safe
(NPO: 164-259 / PBO 930053306)
Office: 082 732 4166
info@staysafe.org.za
neethlingmargaret@gmail.com
www.staysafe.org.za
facebook: staysafewomensroadshow

Stay Safe is a registered NPO offering community-based, self-protection and empowerment training for girls and women. The Stay Safe team consists of eight highly trained and experienced female self-defence practitioners.

Self-Defence Workshops cc
Sanette Smit – Cell: 082 415 3960
Margaret Neethling – Cell: 082 732 4166
P.O. Box 21655, Kloof Street, 8008
smit@selfdefence.co.za or margaret@selfdefence.co.za
facebook: selfdefenceworkshops
www.selfdefence.co.za

Self-Defence Workshops offers a variety of tailored workshops, courses and lectures for corporates, schools, communities and NGOs, as well as specially designed training programmes for provincial and national bodies. Workshops are dynamic, empowering, motivating and highly effective. Standalone safety awareness and empowerment talks can also be booked at your institution or place of work. All workshops are conducted by Sanette Smit, the highest-graded woman in karate in Africa, and include both a practical and theoretical component. These workshops and courses on self-defence and rape prevention are currently the most comprehensive in South Africa.

RAPE COUNSELLING SERVICES/RAPE RESOURCES

CAPE TOWN

Rape Crisis Cape Town Trust (24-hour helpline): 021 447 9762
    Observatory: 021 447 1467
    Athlone: 021 684 1180
    Khayelitsha: 021 361 9228
    Email: communications@rapecrisis.org.za
Lifeline Cape Town: 021 461 1111

PORT ELIZABETH & GRAHAMSTOWN

Rape Crisis Centre: 041 484 3804

DURBAN

Durban Advice Desk for Abused Women: 031 204 4862
Lifeline Durban: 031 312 2323

PRETORIA

Rape Crisis (24-hr number): 082 340 2061
Lifeline Pretoria: 021 342 2222

EAST LONDON

East London Masimanyane Women's Support Centre: 043 743 9169
    Email support: maswsc@iafrica.com
Lifeline East London: 043 722 2000

JOHANNESBURG

People Opposed to Women Abuse (POWA): 011 642 4345/6
Email support: powa1@wn.apc.org

FREE STATE

Lifeline Free State: 057 352 2212

WINDHOEK

Windhoek Women's Solidarity: (09 26461) 26 2275 / (09 26461) 21 5948

NATIONAL NETWORK ON VIOLENCE AGAINST WOMEN

National office: 012 348 1231/3

WEBSITES

www.rape.co.za
www.speakout.org.za
www.rapcan.org.za
www.womensnet.org.za
www.genderstats.org.za

HELPLINES

SAPS Emergency: 10111
Gender-Based Violence Command Centre: 0800 428 428
STOP Gender Violence Helpline: 0800 150 150 / *120*7867#
Halt Elder Abuse Line (HEAL): 0800 003 081

REFERENCES

1. Safe, Secure and Streetwise. 1007, *Reader's Digest*, South Africa.
2. Horos, Carol V.; 1974. *Rape*. Tobey Publishing Co., Inc, Connecticut.
3. Training Manual: *Rape*. 1994, Rape Crisis Cape Town.

4. Levine, Sylvia and Koenig, Joseph; 1983. *Why Men Rape*. W.H. Allen & Co. Ltd, London.
5. Block, Richard and Skogan, Wesley G.; 1986. *Violence and Victims*. Vol. 1, No. 4, Resistance and National Outcomes in Stranger-to-Stranger Predatory Crime.
6. Holmstrom, Lynda Lytle (Ph.D) and Burgess, Ann Wolbert (R.N., D.N. Sc.); 1980. *Archives of Sexual Behaivour*. Vol. 9, No. 5, Sexual Behaivour of Assailants During Reported Rapes.

FURTHER READING

Blundell, Nigel; 1997. *Encyclopaedia of Serial Killers*. PRC, London.
Brownmillar, Susan; 1981. *Against Our Will. Men, Women and Rape*. Bantam Books, U.S.A.
Burgess, Ann Wolbert and Holmstrom, Lynda Lytle; 1979. *Rape, Crisis and Recovery*. Robert J. Brady Co., U.S.A.
Clark, Lorenne and Lewis, Debra; 1977. *Rape: The Price of Coersive Sexuality*. Women's Educational Press, Toronto.
Douglas, John and Olshaker, Mark; 1997. *Mindhunter. Inside the FBI Elite Serial Crime Unit*. Mandarin Paperbacks, London.
Dowdeswell, Jane; 1986. *Women on Rape*. Thorsons Publishing Group, U.K.
Medea, Andra and Thompson, Kathleen; 1984. *Against Rape: A Survival Manual for Women*. McGraw-Hill Ryerson Ltd, Toronto.
Robins, Hoyce and Arnold, Peter; 1994. *Serial Killers: 100 Tales of Infamy, Barbarism and Horrible Crime*. Premier Books, Tyne & Wear.
Russell, Diana E.H.; 1984. *Sexual Exploitation: Rape, Child Sexual Abuse, and Workplace Harassment*. Sage Publications Inc., U.S.A.
Stanko, Elizabeth A.; 1986. *Intimate Intrusions. Women's experience of Male Violence*. Routledge & Kegan Paul Ltd, London.
Vogelman, Lloyd; 1990. *The Sexual Face of Violence. Rapists on rape*. Revan Press (Pty) Ltd, Johannesburg.
Ward, Elizabeth; 1984. *Father Daughter Rape*. Women's Press Limited, London.

www.ingramcontent.com/pod-product-compliance
Lightning Source LLC
Chambersburg PA
CBHW042233090526
44588CB00005B/70